Collins

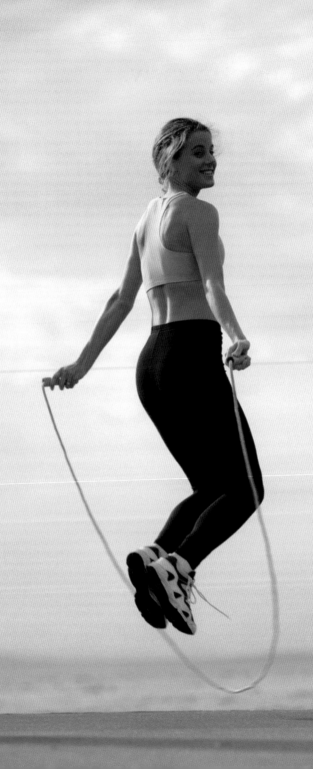

need to know?

How to
Lose
Weight

Christine Michael

Collins

First published in 2006 by Collins
an imprint of
HarperCollins Publishers
77–85 Fulham Palace Road
London W6 8JB

www.collins.co.uk

10 09 08 07 06
6 5 4 3 2 1

A catalogue record for this book is available from
the British Library

Author: Christine Michael
Editor: Heather Thomas
Designer: Rolando Ugolini
Series design: Mark Thomson
Front cover photograph: © Bananastock
Photographs: Charlie Colmer, Rolando Ugolini
Getty Images: pages 7, 11, 15, 36, 40, 137, 147, 166
Rosemary Conley Diet & Fitness Clubs: pages 32, 35,
124, 125, 162
Tables: Scottish Intercollegiate Guidelines Network,
page 13; © Dr Margaret Ashwell, page 18

ISBN-13 978 0 00 720148 8
ISBN-10 0 00 720148 6

Colour reproduction by Colourscan, Singapore
Printed and bound by Great Britain by Butler & Tanner Ltd,Frome

Important
This is a general reference book and although care
has been taken to ensure the information is as
up-to-date and accurate as possible, it is no
substitute for professional advice based on your
personal circumstances. Consult your doctor before
making any major changes to your diet or activity
levels or before taking any over-the-counter
medicines, especially if you have any pre-existing
health problems. Information on specific dieting
methods is provided for reference and should not be
taken as a recommendation or endorsement.

Contents

Introduction

There has never been so much information available to us about healthy eating, weight management and exercise, yet the sheer number of regimes and theories can make it even harder to choose a diet and stick to it. This book will guide you through the weight loss maze, equipping you with the information, confidence and motivation you need to achieve your personal slimming and fitness goals.

A guide for life

Around 13 million adults in the UK are watching their weight or are actively 'on a diet', yet public health statistics suggest this may be a losing battle. Over half of adults are overweight and one in five is at the 'obese' level that represents a significant health risk. So what's going wrong and how can we reverse a trend that suggests that obesity-related diseases will soon overtake smoking as the biggest single cause of premature death?

Beginning with a self-assessment guide to working out your healthy weight range, you will discover the science behind how we lose weight – and put it on – and learn sound healthy-eating principles to ensure that your slimming campaign is safe as well as effective. With so many diets available, there's an assessment of 30 different slimming methods, to help you evaluate all the conflicting information and claims that are made about weight loss products and services. And as getting more active is a vital part of a healthy, slim lifestyle, you'll find a comprehensive guide to boosting fitness and weight loss with the exercise routine that suits you best.

Your chances of success depend on your motivation, confidence and readiness to make the permanent lifestyle changes that are essential to achieving your goal. Find ways to discover your deepest motivations, overcome your inner obstacles and tackle the setbacks that may have led to previous failed attempts at dieting. This book can help you throughout your slimming campaign, providing inspiration, reassurance and support.

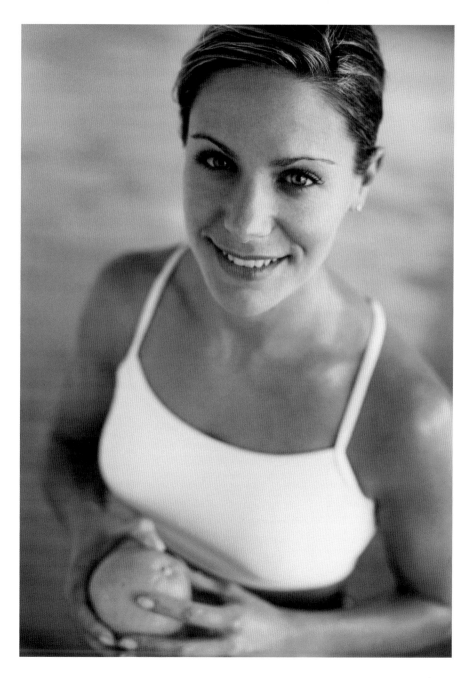

1 The big picture

Before you set yourself a weight loss goal, it is a good idea to find out what kind of shape you are in. These days there is more to working out your ideal weight than just standing on the scales, which only tell part of the story. It takes just a few minutes to discover how healthy your weight and shape are and also to decide what you want to aim for.

Assessing your weight and shape

Do you have a weight problem and, if so, how much do you need to lose to reach the weight range that is healthy for you? Here are some easy ways to find out the facts about your figure.

Measure your BMI
To work out your BMI, you need to divide your weight by your height, squared – a calculator is handy to do the sums.
1 To find your BMI using metric measurements, take your weight in kilograms and your height in metres (get someone to check your height for you if it has been a while).
2 Now divide your weight in kilograms by your height in metres, squared. (To turn your weight in pounds into kilos, divide by 2.2; and to turn inches into metres, multiply by 0.025.)
▶ So if your weight is:
59 kg (9 st 4 lb)
▶ And your height is:
1.6 m (5 ft 4 in)
▶ Your BMI is:
59 ÷ (1.6 x 1.6) = 23.

The scientific approach

Most of us have several different ways of keeping an eye on our weight: for instance, we notice when a favourite pair of trousers feels too tight, or when we do not like what we see in the mirror or on the bathroom scales. To assess what your weight really says about your health and wellbeing though, it pays to take a more scientific approach.

If you've been in denial about your weight for years, the thought of finding out the cold facts might be daunting, but it might not be as bad as you think. Many people have a fixed idea about what their weight 'should be', and often it's based on the slim figure they had as a teenager or on their wedding day, which might not be comfortable or realistic for them now. And if the truth about your weight does come as an unpleasant shock, turn that feeling into a motivational boost. Now that you are about to start a healthy weight loss campaign, you need never see that figure on the scales again.

Body Mass Index

A simple weight-and-height comparison used to be the favoured method of assessing whether someone was overweight or not. Today health professionals prefer to use the Body Mass Index (BMI), a figure that represents your weight per square metre.

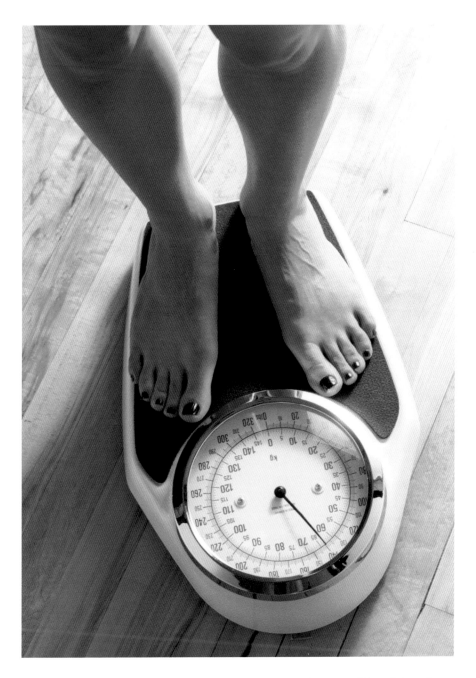

Obesity

Over 20 per cent of British women are obese yet in a Cancer Research survey only four per cent said they were. The health risk starts increasing before it reaches the point where you may look or feel extremely overweight.

Key to the BMI chart

▶ **Colour zone 1**

BMI under 18.5: underweight.
You do not need to lose weight and may even have an increased risk of certain medical conditions that are linked to low body weight, such as osteoporosis ('brittle bones').

▶ **Colour zone 2**

BMI 18.5 – 24.9: normal.
You do not need to lose weight for medical reasons. If you are at the top end of the range, it is worth taking care to eat healthily and exercise regularly to ensure you don't creep into the 'overweight' range.

▶ **Colour zone 3**

BMI 25 – 29.9: overweight.
A BMI of 25-plus indicates that you are over your ideal weight, and in this range you start to increase your risk of developing weight-related health problems. Aiming to lose a few pounds (or more, depending on where you are in the range) will benefit your health.

▶ **Colour zone 4**

BMI 30 – 39.9: obese.
Within this range you are probably at least 14 kg (30 lb) or more over your ideal healthy weight and are running a 'moderate' risk of weight-related medical conditions. As a starting point, losing 10 per cent of your body weight will considerably reduce this risk. If your BMI is between 35 and 39.9, the risk it could pose to your health is classified as 'severe'. A determined effort to lose weight and lower your BMI is worth making a top priority.

▶ **Colour zone 5**

BMI 40 or over: extremely obese.
If you are within this range, then you are probably already experiencing weight-related symptoms and difficulties. Tackling your weight is important and urgent; see your doctor to discuss the various options and to access specialist advice.

BMI chart

Height (in metres)

1.36	1.40	1.44	1.48	1.52	1.56	1.60	1.64	1.68	1.72	1.76	1.80	1.84	1.88	1.92	1.96	2.0	Weight (in kg)

Height columns are printed at 0.02 m intervals (33 columns from 1.36 to 2.0). Weight rows run from 125 kg (top) down to 42 kg (bottom).

Weight (kg)	BMI values (height 1.36 m → 2.0 m, left → right)
125	68 66 64 62 60 59 57 56 54 53 51 50 49 48 46 45 44 43 42 41 40 39 39 38 37 36 35 35 34 33 32 32 31
124	67 65 63 61 60 58 57 55 54 52 51 50 48 47 46 45 44 43 42 41 40 39 38 38 37 36 35 34 33 33 32 32 31
123	67 65 63 61 60 58 57 55 54 52 51 49 48 47 46 45 43 43 42 41 40 39 38 37 37 36 35 34 33 33 32 31 31
122	66 64 62 61 59 57 56 54 53 51 50 49 48 46 45 44 43 42 41 40 39 39 38 37 37 36 35 35 34 33 32 31 30
121	65 64 62 60 58 57 55 54 52 51 50 48 47 46 45 44 43 42 41 40 39 38 37 36 36 35 34 33 33 32 31 31 30
120	65 63 61 60 58 56 55 53 52 51 49 48 47 46 45 43 43 42 41 40 39 38 37 36 35 35 34 33 33 32 31 31 30
119	64 62 61 59 57 56 54 53 52 50 49 48 47 45 44 43 42 41 40 39 38 37 37 36 35 34 33 33 32 31 31 30 29
118	64 62 60 59 57 55 54 52 51 50 48 47 46 45 44 43 42 41 40 39 38 37 36 36 35 34 33 33 32 31 31 30 29
117	63 61 60 58 56 55 53 52 50 49 48 47 46 44 43 42 41 41 40 39 38 38 37 36 35 34 33 33 32 31 30 30 29
116	61 61 59 58 56 54 53 52 50 49 48 46 45 44 43 42 41 40 39 39 38 37 36 35 34 34 33 32 31 31 30 30 29
115	62 60 59 57 55 54 52 51 50 48 47 46 45 44 43 42 41 40 39 38 37 37 36 35 34 34 33 32 32 31 30 29 29
114	62 60 58 57 55 53 52 51 49 48 47 46 45 44 43 41 41 40 39 38 37 36 36 35 34 34 33 32 32 31 30 29 28
113	61 59 58 56 54 53 51 50 49 48 46 45 44 43 42 41 40 39 38 38 37 36 35 35 34 33 32 32 31 30 29 29 28
112	61 59 57 56 54 53 51 50 48 47 46 45 44 43 42 41 40 39 38 37 36 36 35 34 34 33 32 31 30 29 29 28
111	60 58 57 55 53 52 50 49 48 46 45 44 43 42 41 40 39 39 38 37 36 35 35 34 33 32 32 31 30 29 29 28 27
110	59 58 56 55 53 52 50 49 48 46 45 44 43 42 41 40 39 38 37 36 36 35 34 34 33 32 31 31 30 29 28 28 27
109	59 57 56 54 53 51 50 48 47 46 44 44 43 42 40 39 38 37 37 36 35 34 34 33 32 31 31 30 29 28 28 27
108	58 57 55 54 52 51 49 48 47 45 44 43 42 41 40 39 38 37 36 36 35 34 33 33 32 31 30 30 29 28 28 27
107	58 56 55 53 52 50 49 47 46 45 44 43 42 41 40 39 38 37 36 35 34 34 33 32 32 31 30 30 29 28 27 27 26
106	57 56 54 53 51 50 48 47 46 45 43 42 41 40 39 38 37 36 36 35 34 33 33 32 31 31 30 29 28 28 27 26 26
105	57 55 54 52 51 49 48 47 45 44 43 42 41 40 39 38 37 36 35 35 34 33 32 32 31 30 30 29 28 27 27 26 26
104	56 55 53 52 50 49 47 46 45 44 43 42 41 40 39 38 37 36 35 34 33 33 32 31 31 30 29 29 28 27 27 26 26
103	56 54 53 51 50 48 47 46 45 43 42 41 40 39 38 37 36 36 35 34 33 32 32 31 30 30 29 28 28 27 26 26 25
102	55 54 52 51 49 48 47 45 44 43 42 41 40 39 38 37 36 35 34 34 33 32 31 31 30 29 29 28 27 27 26 25 25
101	55 53 52 50 49 47 46 45 44 42 41 40 39 38 37 36 36 35 34 33 32 32 31 30 30 29 28 28 27 26 26 25 25
100	54 53 51 50 48 47 46 44 43 42 41 40 39 38 37 36 35 34 33 33 32 31 31 30 29 28 28 27 27 26 26 25 25
99	54 52 51 49 48 46 45 44 43 42 40 39 38 37 36 36 35 34 33 32 32 31 30 29 29 28 28 27 26 26 25 25 24
98	53 51 50 49 47 46 44 43 42 41 40 39 38 37 36 35 34 33 33 32 31 30 30 29 28 28 27 26 26 25 25 24
97	52 51 49 48 47 45 44 43 42 41 39 38 37 37 36 35 34 33 32 32 31 30 29 29 28 27 27 26 26 25 24 24
96	52 50 49 48 46 45 44 42 41 40 39 38 37 36 35 34 33 33 32 31 30 30 29 28 28 27 26 26 25 25 24 24
95	51 50 48 47 45 44 43 42 41 39 38 37 37 36 35 34 33 32 31 31 30 29 29 28 27 27 26 25 25 24 24
94	51 49 48 47 45 44 43 41 40 39 38 37 36 35 34 33 33 32 31 30 30 29 28 28 27 26 26 25 25 24 24 23
93	50 49 47 46 44 43 42 41 40 39 38 37 36 35 34 33 32 32 31 30 29 29 28 27 27 26 25 25 24 24 23 23
92	50 48 47 45 44 43 42 40 39 38 37 36 35 34 34 33 32 31 30 30 29 28 28 27 26 26 25 25 24 24 23 23
91	49 48 46 45 44 42 41 40 39 38 37 36 35 34 33 32 32 31 30 29 29 28 27 27 26 26 25 24 24 23 23 22
90	49 47 46 45 43 42 41 40 39 38 37 36 35 34 33 32 31 31 30 29 28 28 27 26 26 25 25 24 23 23 22 22
89	48 47 45 44 43 42 41 39 38 37 36 35 34 33 33 32 31 30 29 29 28 27 27 26 25 25 24 24 23 23 22 22
88	48 46 45 44 42 41 40 39 38 37 36 35 34 33 32 31 31 30 29 28 28 27 26 26 25 25 24 23 23 22 22
87	47 46 44 43 42 41 40 39 38 37 35 34 33 33 32 31 30 29 29 28 27 27 26 25 25 24 23 23 22 22 21
86	46 45 44 43 41 40 39 38 37 36 35 34 33 32 31 31 30 29 28 28 27 26 26 25 24 24 23 23 22 22 21 21
85	46 45 43 42 41 40 39 38 37 35 34 34 33 32 31 30 30 29 28 27 27 26 25 25 24 23 23 22 22 21 21
84	45 44 43 42 40 39 38 37 36 35 34 33 32 31 31 30 29 28 28 27 26 26 25 24 24 23 23 22 22 21 21
83	45 44 42 41 40 39 38 37 36 35 34 33 32 31 30 30 29 28 27 27 26 25 25 24 24 23 22 22 21 21 20
82	44 43 42 41 39 38 37 36 35 34 33 32 31 30 30 29 28 27 27 26 25 25 24 24 23 22 22 21 21 20
81	44 43 41 40 39 38 37 36 35 34 33 32 31 30 29 29 28 27 26 26 25 25 24 23 23 22 22 21 21 20 20
80	43 41 40 39 38 37 36 35 34 33 32 31 30 29 29 28 27 27 26 25 25 24 23 23 22 22 21 21 20 20
79	43 41 40 39 38 37 36 35 34 33 32 31 30 29 28 28 27 26 25 25 24 24 23 23 22 21 21 20 20 19
78	42 41 40 38 37 36 35 34 33 32 31 30 29 28 28 27 26 26 25 24 24 23 23 22 22 21 20 20 19
77	41 40 39 38 37 36 35 34 33 32 31 30 29 28 27 27 26 25 25 24 24 23 22 22 21 21 20 20 19 19
76	41 40 39 38 36 35 34 33 32 31 31 30 29 28 27 26 26 25 24 24 23 23 22 21 21 20 20 19 19 18
75	41 39 38 37 35 34 33 32 31 30 29 28 28 27 26 26 25 24 23 23 22 22 21 20 20 19 19 18
74	40 39 38 37 35 34 33 32 31 30 30 29 28 27 26 26 25 24 23 23 22 21 21 20 20 19 19 18 18
73	39 38 37 36 35 34 33 32 31 30 29 28 27 26 26 25 24 24 23 22 22 21 21 20 19 19 18 18
72	39 38 37 36 34 33 32 31 30 29 28 28 27 26 25 25 24 23 23 22 21 21 20 20 19 19 18 18 17
71	38 37 36 35 34 33 32 31 30 29 28 27 26 25 25 24 24 23 22 22 21 20 20 19 19 18 18 17
70	38 37 35 34 33 32 31 30 29 28 28 27 26 25 24 24 23 23 22 21 21 20 20 19 19 18 18 17
69	37 36 35 34 33 32 31 30 29 28 27 26 25 25 24 24 23 22 22 21 20 20 19 19 18 18 18 17
68	37 36 35 34 33 32 31 30 29 28 27 26 25 24 24 23 22 22 21 21 20 19 19 18 18 17 17
67	36 35 34 33 31 30 29 28 28 27 26 25 24 24 23 23 22 21 21 20 20 19 19 18 18 17 17
66	36 35 34 33 32 31 30 29 28 27 26 25 25 24 23 22 22 21 21 20 20 19 18 18 17 17 16
65	35 34 33 32 30 29 28 27 26 26 25 24 23 23 22 22 21 20 20 19 19 18 18 17 17 16 16
64	35 34 32 31 30 29 28 27 27 26 25 24 23 23 22 21 21 20 20 19 18 18 17 17 16 16 15
63	34 33 32 31 30 29 28 27 26 25 24 23 23 22 22 21 20 20 19 19 18 18 17 17 16 16 15
62	33 32 31 30 29 28 27 26 26 25 24 23 22 22 21 21 20 19 19 18 18 17 17 16 16 15 15
61	33 32 31 30 29 28 27 26 25 24 24 23 22 21 21 20 20 19 19 18 18 17 17 16 16 15 15
60	32 31 30 29 28 27 26 25 25 24 23 22 21 21 20 20 19 19 18 18 17 17 16 16 15 15
59	31 30 29 28 27 26 26 25 24 23 23 22 21 21 20 19 19 18 18 17 17 16 16 16 15 15 14
58	31 30 29 28 27 26 25 24 23 23 22 21 21 20 20 19 18 18 17 17 16 16 16 15 15 14 14
57	31 30 29 28 27 26 25 24 23 22 22 21 20 20 19 19 18 18 17 17 16 16 15 15 14 14
56	30 29 28 27 26 25 24 23 23 22 21 21 20 19 19 18 18 17 17 16 16 15 15 14 14 14
55	30 29 28 27 26 25 24 23 22 22 21 20 20 19 19 18 17 17 16 16 15 15 14 14
54	29 28 27 26 25 24 23 23 22 21 21 20 19 19 18 18 17 17 16 16 15 15 14 14 13 13
53	29 27 26 26 25 24 23 22 22 21 20 20 19 18 18 17 17 16 16 15 15 14 14 13 13
52	28 27 26 25 24 23 23 22 21 20 20 19 18 18 17 17 16 16 15 15 14 14 13 13 13
51	28 27 26 25 24 23 22 21 20 20 19 19 18 18 17 17 16 16 15 15 14 14 13 13 12
50	27 26 25 24 23 22 22 21 20 19 19 18 18 17 17 16 16 15 15 14 14 13 13 13 12
49	26 26 25 24 24 23 22 21 20 19 19 18 17 17 16 16 15 15 14 14 14 13 13 12 12
48	26 25 24 23 23 22 21 20 20 19 18 18 17 17 16 16 15 15 14 14 13 13 13 12 12
47	25 24 24 23 22 21 21 20 19 19 18 17 17 16 16 15 15 14 14 13 13 13 12 12 11
46	24 24 23 22 22 21 20 19 19 18 17 17 16 16 15 15 14 14 14 13 13 12 12 11 11
45	24 23 22 22 21 20 20 19 18 18 17 16 16 15 15 15 14 14 13 13 12 12 11 11 11
44	23 23 22 21 21 20 19 19 18 17 17 16 16 15 15 14 14 13 13 13 12 12 11 11 11
43	23 22 21 21 20 20 19 18 18 17 16 16 15 15 15 14 14 13 13 12 12 11 11 11 10
42	23 22 21 20 20 19 19 18 17 17 16 16 15 15 14 14 13 13 12 12 12 11 11 10

4'6"	7"	8"	9"	10"	11"	5'0"	1"	2"	3"	4"	5"	6"	7"	8"	9"	10"	11"	6'0"	1"	2"	3"	4"	5"	6"	7"

Height (in feet and inches)

Assessing your weight and shape | 13

BMI facts
▶ The standard BMI chart is for adults over 18; ask your GP about BMI for children. BMI is not a suitable measure for pregnant or breastfeeding women.
▶ A high BMI might not mean an unhealthy weight for body builders and athletes, who may have a high proportion of muscle, which weighs more than fat.
▶ The BMI might not be a reliable indicator for elderly or frail people who may have very low muscle mass.
▶ There are many online BMI calculators on health websites, but take an average, as from experience they vary.

BMI is based on the assumption that the difference between people who are the same height, but different weights, generally reflects how much fat they have on their bodies. So for assessing health status, BMI is a more accurate measurement than weight versus height alone, as it takes body composition into account.

What your BMI means
The World Health Organization (WHO) has established that a BMI of between 18.5 and 24.9 is 'normal', by which it means that someone whose BMI is within this range has the least risk of developing weight-related health problems.

A BMI of 25–30 is considered 'overweight', with an increased risk of developing weight-related illnesses, such as certain cancers, heart disease and type 2 diabetes (see page 27). The higher your BMI above this level, the more the risk to your health increases and the more you will benefit by losing weight: losing just five to 10 per cent of your body weight and keeping it off can make a difference, so it's well worth aiming for.

Waist management
Your waist measurement is another important indicator of whether you are in healthy shape or not. This is because research has shown that where we carry any excess weight on the body is just as crucial to our overall health as how much extra we might have.

It appears that too much fat around the stomach, seen as an apple shape or 'beer belly', plays a damaging role in increasing the body's resistance to insulin, which in turn can lead to an increased risk of type 2 diabetes and heart disease.

To work out your BMI accurately, you will have to weigh yourself.

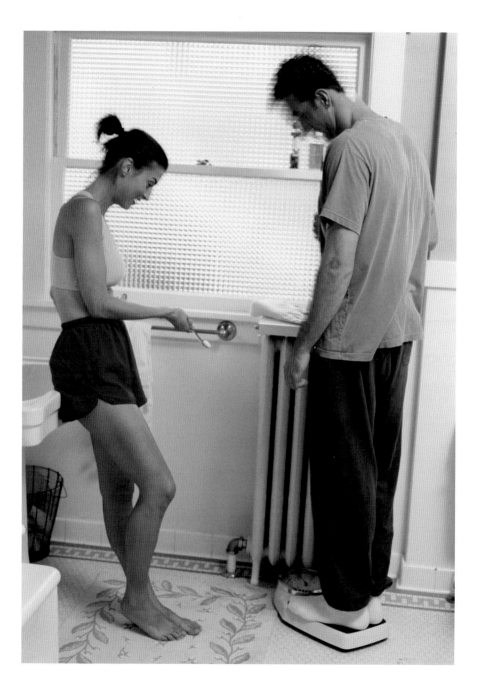

Body fat
An average healthy man has about 15–20 per cent body fat; an overweight man would have about 25 per cent body fat; and an obese man, 35 per cent or more. For women, the figures are 25–27 per cent; 30 per cent; and 35 per cent respectively. You can have your percentage of body fat measured: common methods include skin-fold callipers, bioelectrical impedance or dual energy X-ray absorptiometry.

Going pear-shaped is not bad news for your health.

Someone who is an 'apple' shape will have a greater risk of health problems than someone of the same weight who carries their weight around the hips, thighs and bottom (the classic 'pear' shape).

Measure your waist
To measure your waist, keep the tape measure flat and hold it firmly but not too tightly against your skin. The place to measure is the midpoint between the bottom of the ribs and the top of the hip bone, about 2.5 cm (1 in) above the navel.

Check the table below to see how healthy your waist measurement is. If your BMI is in the normal range but your waist is in the 'increased risk' category, it would be a good idea to lose some weight to slim your waist and stomach.

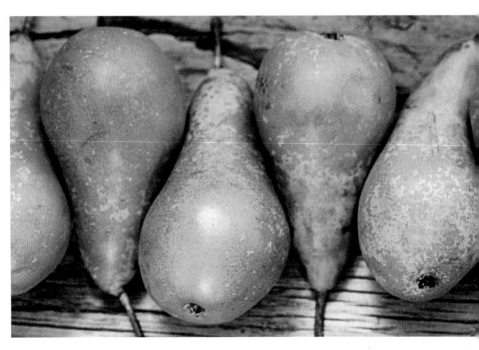

Note: Asian people with 'apple'-shaped waists have been found to be at higher risk of developing health problems than other groups. Asian men with a waist measurement of 90 cm (36 in) or more, and Asian women whose waist is in excess of 80 cm (32 in) are in the 'high risk' group.

How healthy is your waist?

	OK	Increased risk	High risk
Men	94 cm (37 in) or less	94–101 cm (37–39 in)	102 cm (40 in) or more
Women	80 cm (32 in) or less	80–87 cm (32–34 in)	88 cm (35 in) or more

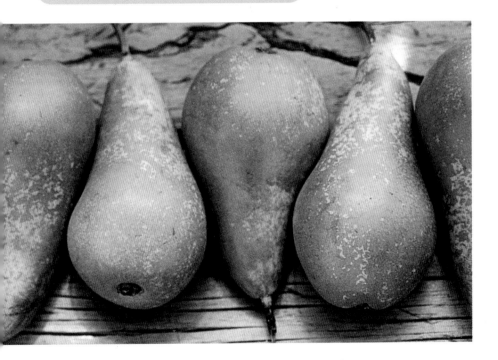

The Ashwell Shape chart

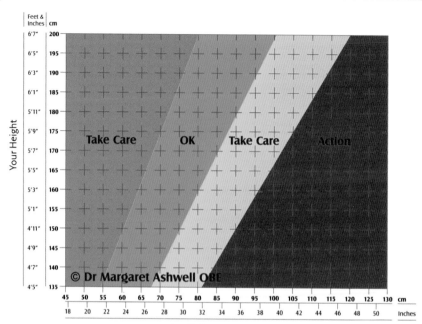

Your Height / Your Waist Measurement

© Dr Margaret Ashwell OBE

▶ **BROWN ZONE**
Your shape suggests you do not need to lose weight and may need to gain it.

▶ **GREEN ZONE**
You have a healthy OK shape.

▶ **AMBER ZONE**
Take care that you don't gain any weight to avoid gaining any inches on your waist and creeping into the 'apple' region.

▶ **RED ZONE**
Your shape indicates that your health is probably at risk. Losing weight will reduce your waist measurement and give a healthier shape.

Does your waist shape up?

The Ashwell Shape Chart (opposite) was developed by leading nutritionist Dr Margaret Ashwell and is an at-a-glance way of checking whether your shape, as determined by your waist and your height, is in a healthy range or not. To use the chart, just read off your height in a horizontal line and your waist measurement in a vertical line. The point where the two lines meet is where your shape is on the chart.

Apple shapes

Fat seems to be more easily lost from 'apple' shapes than from 'pears', and this could help to explain why men often seem to slim more quickly than women. Being stressed stimulates production of the hormone cortisol, which is known to play a part in distributing stored fat in the central abdominal area, and this could contribute to an 'apple' shape. Fat stored in the central area is found deep down in the region of the stomach, while fat on the hips, thighs and bottom is stored nearer the surface of the skin. This can give it the 'orange peel' texture known as cellulite, so it is a small consolation that while it may not look attractive, it is less harmful to health than central abdominal fat.

Quick measures

▶ If you can pinch more than an inch of fat at the back of your upper arm or at your midriff, you're probably overweight.
▶ Another method is to divide your hip measurement by your waist measurement: if the result is less than 1, you are a 'pear'; if it's more than 1, you are an 'apple'.
▶ If your waist measurement is less than half your height, your shape is likely to be in the 'OK' healthy range.

want to know more?

Take it to the next level...

▶ **Your weight and health** 22
▶ **Cellulite** 113
▶ **Assessing your fitness level** 149
▶ **Increasing exercise** 134

Other sources
▶ **Gyms and health spas may offer body composition tests which tell you the percentage of body fat, water and lean tissue in your body.**
▶ **Book in for a lifestyle 'MOT' at your local surgery to test for weight-related conditions.**
▶ **Invest in the latest bathroom scales that measure BMI and body fat percentage as well as your weight.**
▶ **Join a fitness class to tone up troublesome areas such as your stomach, bottom and thighs.**
▶ **For books on fitness training and exercise, see page 189.**
▶ **For more on the Ashwell Shape Chart, see www.ashwell.uk.com**

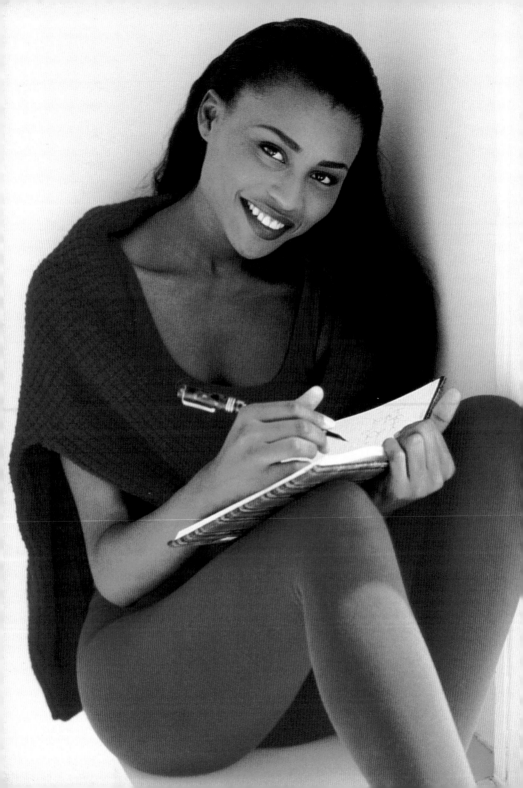

2 Healthy weight, healthier you

Taking care of your weight is one of the most important things that you can do to maximize your chances of living a long and healthy life. The good news is that if you are overweight, you don't need to slim down to a 'perfect' size in order to reap the health benefits – every pound that you lose can help, which is great motivation to get started.

Why overweight is a big deal

Carrying excess weight means increasing the risk of health problems, either as a direct result of being heavier or from the likelihood of developing diseases in later life. Being aware of this is the first step to feeling more in control of your weight and your health.

must know

Stop smoking

Smoking is a bigger hazard to health than being overweight, yet some people – especially women – smoke to help keep their weight down. Giving up smoking does not mean you will automatically put on weight but weight gains of 1.8–3.2 kg (4–7 lb) are common; this seems to be because food tastes better and people snack more rather than any physiological reason. Trying to stop smoking and lose weight at the same time is a big job. Tackle smoking first, aiming to minimize any weight gain by eating healthily and being as active as possible – and then make your weight a priority.

Awareness, not worry

Good health would be top of most people's list of ingredients for a happy life, and in an ideal world, we would choose to avoid illness and disability if we possibly could. In the real world, of course, we have to play with the cards that life deals us, and many of the factors that determine our long-term health are beyond our control.

However, that does not mean that we should not try to change the odds in our favour whenever we can do so. The overwhelming evidence, from scientific research that has been carried out around the world, is that managing our weight is one of the optimum ways to give ourselves the best possible chance of living a long, healthy and active life.

Consumer studies suggest, however, that improving their health is not always the main reason why people start a diet or fitness regime. About half of slimmers, especially younger ones, say that they want to lose weight in order to look better in clothes, or for a special occasion such as a forthcoming holiday or wedding. And that's absolutely fine!

It is fantastic to know that you look your best, and to be able to wear whatever you want and to enjoy looking at your holiday photos instead of dreading them.

All too often, for health to become the main motivator to embark on a slimming regime it takes a crisis: perhaps your doctor warns that your blood pressure is too high, or recommends you lose weight before trying for a baby, or you find that you are increasingly breathless and uncomfortable.

But health can be a positive motivator as well as a cause of fear and worry. Skim through this section, and you will see that while some of the health implications of being overweight are serious, it does not take a massive weight loss to reduce your risk of developing problems, or to improve symptoms that might be bothering you already. If you only have a little weight to lose, knowing that you are benefitting your health by reaching and maintaining your target weight can be a deep source of satisfaction – in addition to the joys of shopping for smaller clothes.

Facts of life

Can you be overweight and healthy? The answer is yes – and no. Of course your overall health depends on many risk factors, such as your family history, whether you smoke or drink heavily, your fitness level, where you carry your weight and so on. If being overweight is your only risk factor, then you have more chance of remaining in good health than someone who ticks a lot of 'risk' boxes. And there will always be overweight people who reach a hale and hearty old age without losing a pound.

Unfortunately, however, statistics show that if you are overweight you are unlikely to be one of those people – they are the exception that proves the rule. Here are five disturbing facts, which come from UK National Health Service-endorsed studies:

▶ If your BMI is 24 or more, your risk of dying within a 26-year period increases by one per cent for every pound put on between the ages of 30 and 42, and by two per cent for every pound gained between the ages of 50 and 62.

▶ Deaths linked to obesity, of which there are about 30,000 a year, shorten the life of the deceased by nine years on average.

▶ Your risk of coronary heart disease doubles at a BMI of over 25, and nearly quadruples at a BMI of 29 or more.

▶ The risk of developing type 2 diabetes is 40 times greater at a BMI of 35 or more.

▶ Ill health linked to obesity is responsible for 18 million days off work a year and costs the NHS at least £500 million a year in treatment.

Why weight is to blame

It is easy to imagine why being overweight can cause certain health problems – breathlessness or pain in weight-bearing joints such as the knees and lower spine. Some medical conditions, however, have a more complex relationship with weight. As we saw earlier, a BMI of between 18.5 and 24.9 is thought to be within the desirable 'healthy' range, so, in theory, any weight gain that takes your BMI above 25 is potentially a risk to your health. It is generally accepted though that the risk of serious conditions, such as diabetes and heart disease, rises significantly at a BMI of around 27 or above.

So why worry if you are only a few pounds overweight? The trouble is that extra pounds can have a habit of creeping up on us unawares. So if your BMI hovers around the 25 level, it makes sense to keep your weight stable or to lose a few pounds. And, of course, if your BMI is unhealthily high, slimming will quickly bring big benefits (see page 29).

Weight-related health problems

Below is some background information to the most common weight-related health problems that may develop.

Make the most of seasonal food like berries to give your health a boost.

Coronary heart disease

One of the key aspects of heart health is the ability of the heart and its surrounding arteries to circulate blood strongly and freely

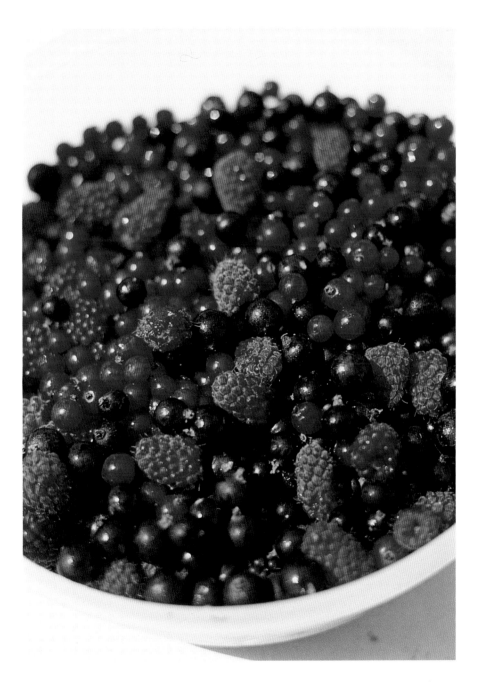

Change the odds on good health in your favour by eating well.

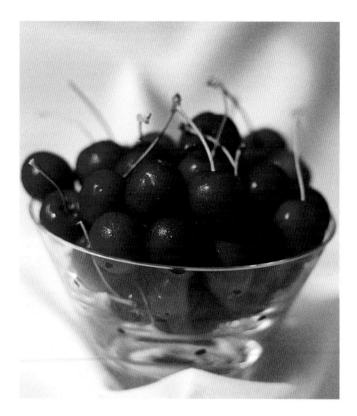

must know

Body fat
This is not always the bad guy! We need a certain amount of body fat to protect and insulate our organs; it also has a role in producing certain beneficial hormones, and protects against loss of bone mass (osteoporosis).

round the body. Being overweight can damage heart health in a number of ways, mainly by raising the level of unhealthy fats, such as low-density lipoprotein (LDL) cholesterol and triglycerides, in the blood. A build-up of these fats over time can narrow or clog the arteries, a condition known as atherosclerosis, and this in turn can lead to chronic diseases such as angina, or acute conditions such as a heart attack.

High blood pressure, which is three times more common among overweight people than slim people, is also a big risk factor. And even where there are no problems with blood fats or blood pressure, just carrying excess weight, especially around the middle, seems to increase the likelihood of developing heart disease.

Type 2 diabetes

This condition affects 1.4 million people in the UK and possibly a further million who have not had their condition diagnosed, according to the charity Diabetes UK. Type 2 diabetes is sometimes called 'late onset' because, unlike type 1, it tends to develop in adult life, and being overweight is a big risk factor: over 80 per cent of adults with type 2 diabetes have a BMI of more than 25 when they are diagnosed. Children and teenagers are also being diagnosed more frequently as obesity rises.

Type 2 diabetes is caused when the insulin that the pancreas produces in the body fails to control blood sugar properly (insulin resistance) or when the pancreas fails to produce enough insulin for the body's needs. Research shows that excess weight, especially around the waistline, increases insulin resistance so the pancreas has to work harder to get the same effect. Having too much sugar in the blood causes symptoms such as excessive thirst, blurred vision, fatigue and passing urine frequently. Having too much insulin in the blood causes other problems, such as increasing blood pressure and raising the level of various fats in the blood. This puts people with type 2 diabetes at high risk of heart disease and stroke; untreated diabetes can also cause serious damage to the eyes, kidneys, nerves and circulation.

Cancers

Cancer Research UK states that after smoking, obesity is the second biggest preventable cause of cancers. The links between being overweight and cancer are complex and not all of them are fully understood.

must know

'Syndrome X'
Also known as metabolic syndrome, this term refers to a collection of symptoms that include evidence of insulin resistance, fat carried around the middle ('apple' shape), high blood pressure and raised levels of unhealthy fats (LDL cholesterol and triglycerides) in the blood. Together, they represent an increased risk of heart disease, diabetes or stroke. Some diets claim to have specific benefits for people with Syndrome X, but any healthy eating and exercise programme, leading to a five or 10 per cent initial weight loss, should reduce all these symptoms without any special diets being needed.

Weight reduction benefits
Here is an overview of the
average benefits of a 10 per
cent (10 kg or 22 lb) reduction in
weight of a man with a starting
weight of 100 kg (220 lb) or just
under 16 stone.
▶ The risk of premature death
is reduced by 25 per cent.
▶ Systolic blood pressure is
down by 10 points, and dystolic
blood pressure down by
20 points.
▶ The level of LDL cholesterol
is down by 15 per cent.
▶ The risk of dying from
diabetes complications is
down by 30-40 per cent.
▶ The risk of dying from obesity-
related cancer is reduced by
40-50 per cent.

However, it seems that obesity can unbalance the
function of certain hormones, which could increase
the risk of hormonally-sensitive cancers in women,
such as cancer of the uterus, ovaries, cervix and
endometrium (uterus lining). Excess abdominal fat
(the 'apple' shape) has also been linked to a higher
risk of breast cancer in women after the menopause.
Cancers of the digestive system, such as colon or
rectal cancer, may have more of a link to a high-fat,
low-fibre diet, which is likely to lead to weight gain.

High blood pressure
Blood pressure is measured by taking two readings:
the systolic pressure (the first, higher figure, taken
when the heart contracts) and the dystolic pressure
(the second, lower pressure, taken when the heart
is relaxed). A normal level is 120/80, and a reading
that is consistently over 140/90 is unhealthily high.
Many people with high blood pressure have no
symptoms, but that does not necessarily mean that
there is no problem: untreated high blood pressure
can cause a stroke, heart disease or damage to other
organs in the body.

Being overweight is not the only cause of high
blood pressure: eating too much salt, drinking
too much alcohol and being inactive can also
contribute. The good news is that as well as losing
weight, changing your diet and lifestyle is a quick
and effective way to reduce your blood pressure.

Gall bladder disease
One large study found that overweight women were
33 per cent more likely to develop gallstones than a
similar group of healthy-weight women. Gallstones

are a painful side-effect of the build-up of fats in the blood, as they are caused by clumps of cholesterol in the gall bladder, which plays a part in digestion. Cancer of the gall bladder is a rarer complication.

You lose, you win!

As we said at the beginning of this chapter, knowing the facts about the serious health consequences of being overweight is not all bad news. The flipside of the problems of gaining weight is that losing weight can bring quick and significant health benefits. A reassuring body of research has concluded that if you are seriously overweight (BMI of 30 or more), then losing just 10 per cent of your body weight can improve your health and even add years to your life.

Other health benefits

As well as the established evidence of improvements to these life-threatening aspects of obesity, successful slimmers often report that losing weight benefits their health and wellbeing in many other ways, too. These can include improving the symptoms of asthma; less heavy or painful periods; reducing backache, arthritis pain and gout; improving digestive conditions such as irritable bowel syndrome; getting a better night's sleep (being seriously overweight can lead to a distressing and dangerous condition called obstructive sleep apnoea); and a general lifting of mood.

Add to all these benefits the overall feel-good factor that comes from having more energy, feeling fitter and healthier, and experiencing the confidence that comes from knowing that you are looking good. It is hardly surprising that people who have lost weight successfully nearly always say: 'I just wish I'd done it sooner.'

want to know more?

Take it to the next level...

▶ **Cutting down on salt** 60
▶ **Diabetes and the Glycaemic Index** 98
▶ **Slimming clubs** 124
▶ **Energy and fitness** 134
▶ **Maintaining a healthy weight** 168

Other sources
▶ **Consult your doctor if you have any symptoms of diabetes.**
▶ **Check your blood pressure; many people don't know that theirs is too high.**
▶ **If you are very overweight, see your GP or practice nurse about slimming strategies. Some offer free or low-cost referral to local slimming clubs or leisure centres, for extra support.**
▶ **For help on quitting smoking, call the NHS Smoking Helpline on 0800 169 0 169. www.quit.org.uk**
▶ **For advice on eating disorders, contact the Eating Disorders Association helpline: 0845 634 1414. www.edauk.com**

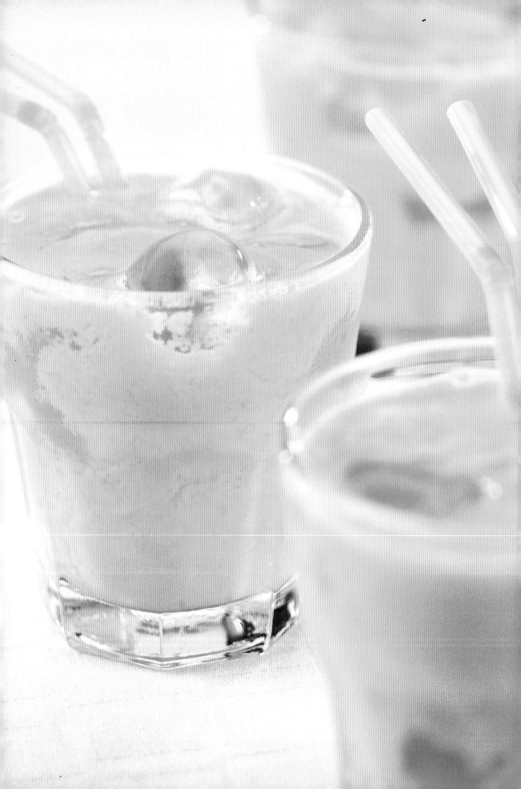

3 In search of a cause

As a nation, we are gaining weight faster than ever before in our history and obesity is now officially classed as an epidemic. How can this be happening? Is it 'all in our genes', or are our modern diet and environment to blame? The truth is complex but one thing is clear: being aware of the theories can help you to find your own practical solution.

Why we're the shape we're in

Why do some people put on weight easily while others seem to eat what they like and stay slim? We don't fully understand but the evidence has a positive message: in health and fitness, nearly all of us have the power to take our destiny into our own hands.

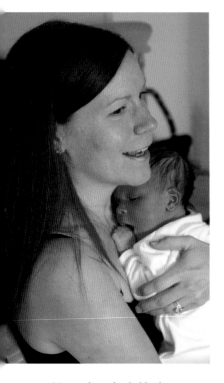

It's worth getting babies into healthy eating habits as early as possible: overweight children are more likely to stay that way into adult life.

The energy equation

There is no getting away from it: we gain weight when we eat more calories than we expend, and vice versa. This 'energy equation' is a basic law of physics and it is important not to lose sight of it, especially if you are weighing up some of the commercial weight-loss plans on offer. Any diet that promises that you can slim without changing your diet or activity level in any way is one to strike off your list!

However, the simple truth of the energy equation hides a multitude of complex factors that can affect, on the one side, how and why we eat, and on the other, how efficiently our bodies burn fuel. These factors include our genetic make-up; our age; our metabolism; our environment; our state of general health; and our emotional response to food.

Very often you will read about a new scientific breakthrough that appears to lay the blame for our weight problems solely at the door of one of these factors: 'it's all in our genes' or 'how hormones make you fat'. In reality, however, it is unlikely that any single discovery will ever give us all the answers or provide a complete solution. And in a way this is good news because it means that we have more control than we might think over the many factors that affect our weight, and there is a lot that we can do to improve our chances of staying in good shape throughout our lives.

Family matters

A child with two obese parents has a 70 per cent chance of becoming obese, compared to 20 per cent for a child of two slim parents. That alone suggests strongly that our weight is predetermined by what we inherit from our parents. But how far is that inheritance down to genes, and how much is due to the family's lifestyle? And if the link is genetic, which side of the energy equation are the inherited genes affecting?

Much of the current research into the link between genes and weight concerns the behaviour of individual genes and how they affect our appetite or the way we turn food into energy. There have been some exciting developments: for instance, it has been shown that in very rare cases, severe obesity is caused by a genetic mutation that causes the failure of a hormone called leptin, which regulates appetite in the brain. Children born without leptin will eat uncontrollably, but their appetite and weight will return to normal once they receive leptin injections.

Our caveman inheritance

Eventually, research into leptin deficiency and some other specific gene mutations may lead to effective treatments for what scientists now call 'common obesity'. However, whereas only a very few people are unlucky enough to have faulty genes, none of us can escape the genetic pattern that has been handed down to us over millions of years.

Getting heavier?
There is now evidence that our environment can seriously damage our size. In 1955, fewer cars and more housework meant that the average woman could expend up to 800 calories a day more in activity than she does today. According to a recent survey, the average woman now weighs 65 kg (10 st 3.5 lb) and measures 38–34–40.5, but in 1951 she weighed 62 kg (9 st 10 lb) and she measured 37–27.5–39.

Our earliest human ancestors evolved in an
environment where food supplies were scarce
and sporadic. Our strongest food preferences and
cravings – for sweet, fatty and salty foods – are a
reminder of the times when sources of glucose,
essential fats and minerals were hard to come by.
Energy conservation in time of famine was vital, so
those human beings who had 'thrifty genes' – who
were most able to convert food to fat and store it
effectively – were the most likely to survive, breed
and pass on those genes.

Old genes, new environment
Unfortunately, the genetic make-up that suited
us so well for survival in prehistoric times is very
unhelpful today in our modern environment.
Instead of eating fatty, sweet or salty foods only
rarely, we now have access to them 24 hours a day,
seven days a week, if we want. When we do eat
excess fat and sugar, our 'thrifty genes' ensure that
we store it very efficiently as fat. And instead of
foraging and hunting to find our food, we only have
to drive to the supermarket, pick up the phone or
log on to the internet.

So how can a history lesson help us to lose
weight? One vital thing it teaches us is that weight
is not a moral issue. People do not put on weight
because they are essentially greedy, lazy or sinful:
on the contrary, gaining weight is the natural
human response to life in a food-rich and activity-
poor environment. If our ancestors had had the
choice between hunting for their food or going to
the supermarket, which one do you think they
would have chosen?

From generation to generation,
it's hard for us to escape the
genetic patterns that are handed
down through the ages.

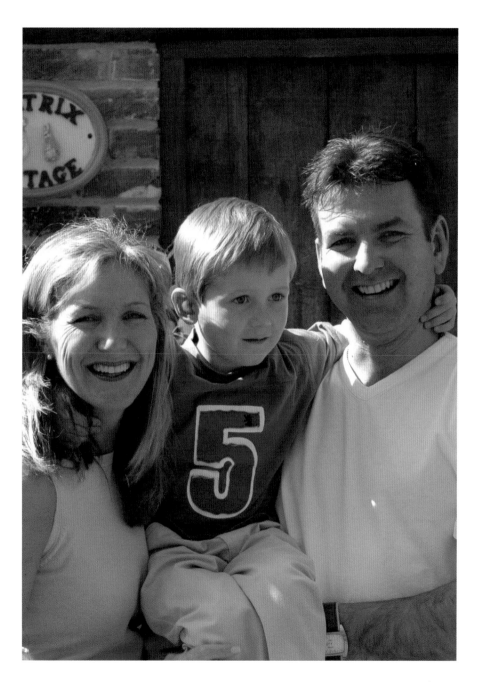

As we are discovering, the fact that our genes have not yet caught up with our environment is bad news for our health. So the other lesson that history teaches us is that, as we cannot change our genes, in order to stay slim and healthy we need to adapt our environment – with small changes to diet and lifestyle that can swing the energy balance back in our favour.

Metabolism

This is the process by which the body converts the food that we eat into everything it needs to function, and as such it plays a key role in regulating

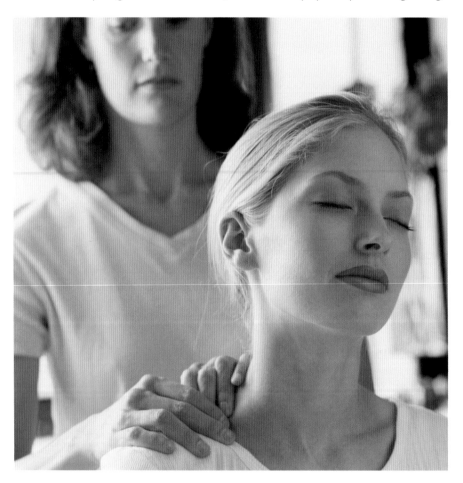

our weight. Between 20 and 30 per cent of the energy that our metabolism produces is spent on exercise, and between five and 10 per cent is used to digest our food. The remaining energy – which is between 60 and 75 per cent – is consumed as 'resting metabolic expenditure' (RME), and this can vary widely between individuals. Medical problems that can affect the metabolism include an under-active thyroid and, in very rare cases, conditions such as Prader-Willi Syndrome.

must know

Fast food
It's official: fast food causes weight gain. A 15-year study in the US showed that people who ate at fast food restaurants more than twice a week gained an extra 4.5 kg (10 lb) compared to those who ate fast food less than once a week.

People with weight problems often believe they have a slow metabolism, but in fact overweight people have a faster metabolism than average as they need to burn energy more efficiently to move a heavier body around. This explains why slimmers often find it hard to lose the last few pounds towards their target; with less weight to carry, the body requires slightly fewer calories to support the metabolic process and therefore their diet and exercise plan might need a slight adjustment. This does not mean though that dieting 'damages' the metabolism; it is a natural process that re-sets the body's energy balance over time.

One major factor that influences your metabolic rate though is the amount of lean muscle tissue in your body, as lean tissue is a more efficient fuel-burner than fat. Becoming more active is a great way to boost your metabolism – exercise burns fat, and builds muscle, which burns fat more efficiently... a win-win situation for your body.

A NEAT trick

Scientists are also excited about the way that we move and use energy when we're not consciously exercising: a process they call Non-Exercise Activity Thermogenesis (NEAT). Studies at the Mayo Clinic in Minnesota, USA, have shown that obese people expend fewer calories in all areas of daily life than slim people; they sit still for longer periods and even fidget less. Researchers estimate that slim people could 'naturally' burn up to 350 calories more per day

If you're stressed, try to relax or have a massage rather than comfort eating.

in this way than overweight people – the equivalent of a 30-minute run. When slim volunteers were overfed so that they put on weight, their energy output remained the same, however, suggesting that the overweight people were not being 'lazy': there is a bio-chemical process at work that predisposes them to be less active.

While it may take years to identify exactly how and why this happens, it is further evidence that making activity an everyday habit is key to losing weight and staying slim – wherever you start on the road from completely sedentary to fighting fit.

Eating for two

A 2005 survey of 2,000 new mothers found that nearly two years after giving birth, their average weight was a stone heavier than they had been before their pregnancy. Of course, putting on some weight is expected and desirable in pregnancy. However, many women who have never had a weight problem find that the pounds pile on and then prove very hard to lose long after their baby is born – so much so that they despair that pregnancy has somehow changed their natural weight forever. The reassuring news is that there seems to be no fundamental, physical reason why this should be the case. It appears more likely that any weight gain is a side-effect of the upheaval in lifestyle that can come with the arrival of a new baby: lack of sleep, snatched meals, no time for exercise and more time spent at home can all alter the energy balance sufficiently so that weight goes on and stays put.

Monitoring your weight in pregnancy and not 'eating for two' so that you do not gain too much is sensible; around 13 kg (28 lb) is an average amount. Breastfeeding is good for the baby and for you, as it uses up around 500 calories a day. Crash diets and intensive exercise are not the way to regain your pre-pregnancy shape, whatever you might read

must know

Drugs and medication
Weight gain can be a side-effect of some drugs and medical treatments. These include cancer drugs, such as tamoxifen; some steroids and antidepressants; and some drugs for diabetes and epilepsy. Ask your GP about the side-effects of any medication you are prescribed and whether you need to be careful about your diet while you are taking it.

in celebrity magazines. Instead, go for a slow and steady weight loss, with a healthy diet and gradual increase in activity, and aim to lose any surplus pounds over a period of months rather than weeks.

It's my age

Is it inevitable to gain weight as we get older? Surveys suggest that we are at our heaviest in our 40s and 50s, and that the main reason for this is that we become gradually less active, rather than eating more. One large research project found that most adults will gain 9 kg (20 lb) between the ages of 20 and 55 years unless they take specific steps to avoid it.

So eating as if you are still playing football twice a week, when these days you are watching it on television twice a week, is a relatively effective way to score an own-goal as far as your weight goes.

The menopause

Women going through the menopause often feel they have more trouble managing their weight and may accept gaining the 'menopause 10' as an inevitable side-effect. However, as with pregnancy, that other major hormonal event, research suggests that the menopause does not necessarily lead directly to weight gain, although increased levels of testosterone and decreased levels of oestrogen may mean that the distribution of weight will change slightly, so that 'pear' shapes become 'apples' – the classic middle-age spread.

As we saw earlier, carrying excess weight around the waist represents a higher risk of developing health problems than on the hips and thighs, so it is well worth aiming to get your weight into the healthy range and your waist below 80 cm (32 in).

want to know more?

Take it to the next level...

▶ **Work out your own energy balance** 46
▶ **Boost your metabolism with exercise** 138
▶ **Build activity into daily life** 144

Other sources

▶ **Buy a pedometer to monitor how active you are each day.**
▶ **Swap to low-fat, low-sugar versions of the foods you crave to enjoy the taste without the calories.**
▶ **For more on healthy family eating: www.nutrition.org.uk**
▶ **Spot the obesogens in your daily life: are there ways to combat them?**
▶ **Join a reputable slimming club for support in healthy eating and managing your weight.**

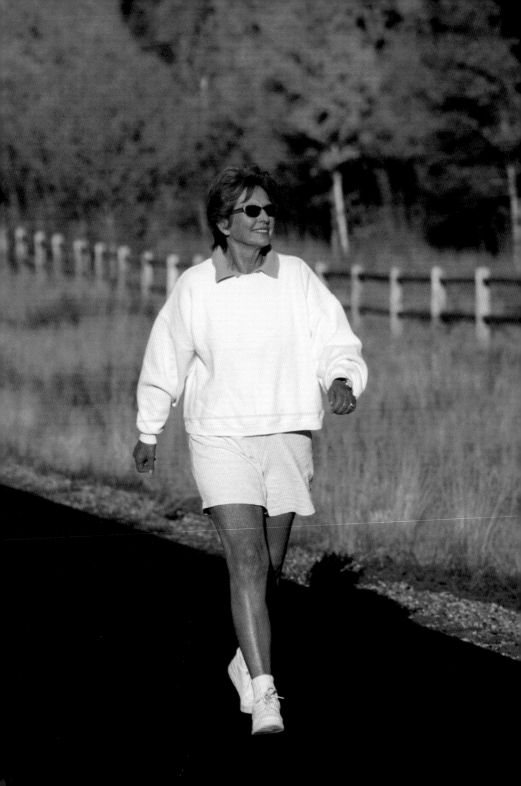

4 The science of weight loss

Understanding the energy equation and how to alter it in order to promote weight loss instead of weight gain is the key to reaching a healthy weight. Knowing the facts can be the basis of taking control of your weight and staying motivated throughout a safe and steady weight loss campaign.

The energy balance

The last section looked at the energy equation and the different factors that can affect it. Now the time has come to apply those principles to individual circumstances.

Altering the energy balance

The next few pages set out how far to reduce your calorie intake and increase your calorie output in order to create your own personalized slimming plan which will guarantee safe and steady weight loss.

As the previous chapter showed, the science behind weight loss and weight gain is all about the energy equation: consuming more energy, in the form of food, than is expended in activity results in weight gain. To lose weight, it is essential to create an 'energy deficit' so that more energy is expended in activity than is taken into the body as food.

Units of energy

The units of energy used to measure this process are kilojoules or calories – the word that can be very off-putting for people who have followed the kind of diet that requires the counting and measuring of every single mouthful they consume. Unfortunately, it is impossible to ignore calories when trying to lose weight. It is true that there are plenty of diets that promise you 'need never count another calorie'. This is generally because they either give calories another name, such as 'units', or because they ensure that calorie intake is controlled automatically by limiting the kinds of foods that can be eaten.

Calculating your energy deficit

The aim of this section is to show you how to calculate a personalized energy deficit by working out:

▶ Your current energy expenditure.
▶ Your current energy consumption.
▶ Your daily energy requirements needed to lose weight steadily.

Inevitably, this means talking about calories. However, it is possible to lose weight easily by being calorie-conscious and without having to become a calorie slave.

Bulky, watery foods like salad vegetables make good low-calorie fillers in a slimming diet.

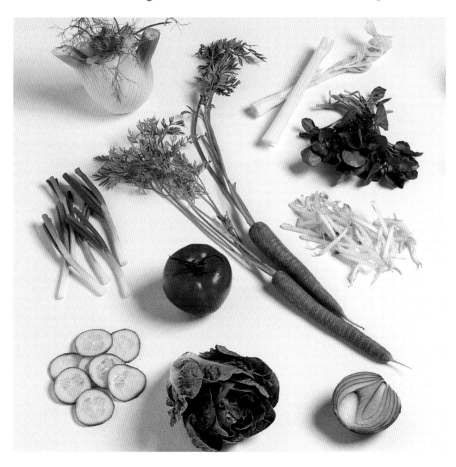

must know

Diet or exercise?
When thinking about losing weight, men and women tend to have different approaches: women say it's 'time to start the diet' and men say it's 'time to hit the gym'. It is perfectly possible to create an energy deficit by changing your diet alone, or just by doing a lot more exercise (although the exercise-only route is slower). The perfect combination for health and weight loss is to do both: to make some small changes to your diet, and to become a bit more active as often as possible.

Where does it all go?

The body uses the food we eat in three main ways: for growth; to replace damaged or worn-out tissues; and to fulfil all the body's daily functions, which can range from breathing to ballroom dancing. The amount of energy needed from food to keep the body going, without gaining or losing weight, is called the basal metabolic rate (BMR). Any energy (calories) which is taken in over and above the requirements of the BMR is stored – and, as the last chapter showed, this is one thing at which the body is very efficient.

Once food has been digested, any surplus energy is stored either as glycogen – a short-term energy source, which is stored in the liver and the muscles – or as fat, which is stored in 'fat depots' under the skin, around the kidneys and in the abdomen. There is a limit as to how much glycogen can be stored before it is released back into the bloodstream to be used, but there is no limit to the amount of fat that can be stored. Fat cells get bigger, multiply and form adipose tissue which can eventually present a threat to our health.

It takes about 3,500 calories surplus to the requirements of the BMR to create 1lb (454 g) of stored energy (otherwise known as fat). So an individual whose BMR is 2,500 calories per day, and who eats 3,000 calories' worth of food per day without changing his or her activity level in any way, could expect to put on a pound a week (7 x 500 = 3,500 calories). In practice, our body weight fluctuates from day to day and even at different times of the day, which is why it is best to weigh yourself only once a week at the same time – jumping on the scales more often can be misleading. However, over time, a steady over-supply of calories without an increase in activity to compensate will surely result in a weight gain.

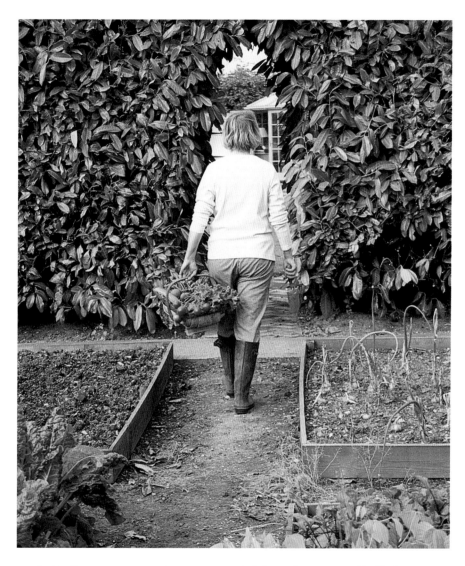

And in the same way, creating an energy deficit, so that more energy is expended than the BMR requires, will equally surely result, over time, in weight loss. So, again, someone whose BMR is 2,500 calories and who eats 2,000 calories' worth of food each day could expect to lose a pound a week.

Healthy home-grown vegetables: fantastic for taste, freshness and providing valuable nutrients.

Find your balance

There are four steps to working out your basal metabolic rate (BMR):

1 Assessing the resting metabolic expenditure (RME).

2 Making an allowance for activity.

3 Adding in 10 per cent for the energy used in digesting food.

4 Totalling it all up.

As you will see from the instructions and the example given below, this is much easier than it sounds.

Step 1

Use the table to read off your RME. The differences in the table are accounted for by gender and age: generally, men need more calories than women to maintain their weight because they have a higher percentage of muscle tissue, which burns fuel more efficiently than fat. Age is a factor, too, because the amount of energy the body needs for maintenance peaks at the age of about 25 and declines gradually after that, at a rate of about two per cent per decade.

Your RME

Age – Men	RME equation
18 – 30	15.3 x weight (kg) + 679
30 – 60	11.6 x weight (kg) + 879
60 and above	13.5 x weight (kg) + 487

Age – Women	RME equation
18 – 30	14.7 x weight (kg) + 496
30 – 60	8.7 x weight (kg) + 829
60 and above	10.5 x weight (kg) + 596

Step 2

Factor in your activity level, based on what you normally spend most of the day doing. The guidelines and calculation are as in the table opposite (top).

Multiply your RME from Step 1 by the activity factor to find the number of calories needed for activity each day.

Your activity level

Usual daily activities	Activity Level	Activity Factor
Desk job or light housework; driving; reading; watching TV	Very light	0.2
Childcare; light exercise, e.g. walks; moderate housework; light manual work, e.g. mechanic, waiter	Light	0.3
Moving about all day; spring-cleaning; heavy gardening; active sports	Moderate	0.4
Heavy manual work, e.g. building, digging; high-energy sport, e.g. football	Heavy	0.5

Step 3

Add together your RME figure and your 'activity calories' figure and divide by 10 to find the calories needed for digestion.

Step 4

Add together your RME figure, 'activity calories' figure and 'digestion calories' figure in order to find your BMR (basal metabolic rate) – the total number of calories that are needed each day to maintain your weight.

To lose weight steadily, the best combination is to reduce your calorie intake and to increase your calorie expenditure by making changes to your daily diet and activity levels.

must know

Working out BMR
Jane is a 30-year-old mother of two with a part-time office job. She weighs 76 kg (12 stone).
▶ In step 1, Jane works out her RME to be:
$8.7 \times 76 + 829 = 1,490$ calories.
▶ In step 2, she estimates her activity level as 'light' and her activity factor as 0.3. So the calories she needs for activity are:
$1,490 \times 0.3 = 447$
▶ In step 3, Jane adds her RME and activity calories together and divides by 10 to find the calories she needs for digestion:
$1,490 + 447 = 1,937 \div 10 = 193$
▶ In step 4, she adds the three totals together to find her BMR (total daily calorie needs):
$1,490 + 447 + 193 = 2,130$ calories.

must know

Calorie savings
Look over your
food diary to
identify the areas
where it would
be easy for you
to make calorie
savings.

Keeping a food diary

Having worked out how many calories you need to maintain
your current weight, the next step is to work out how many
calories you are taking in as food. Nutritionists recommend
that the best way to do this is to keep a food diary. To get a
full picture of calorie intake it is important to keep the diary
for at least a week, or longer if you feel it would be helpful.
Keeping a food diary sounds easy but, in practice, researchers
have found that people who are asked to record their food
intake almost always under-report what they actually eat.
However, to identify patterns of where calories are coming from
and where easy savings can be made, it is important to be as
detailed and honest as possible – after all, no one else will see
the diary. It is also important to eat and drink exactly as usual
and not to change your normal routine in any way, as you need
to keep track of all the occasions during the week when you
might have an opportunity to save calories.

Sample food diary for a single day

Breakfast
Med egg, 2 rashers back bacon, 1 tbsp vegetable oil, 2 slices white toast,
2 tsp butter, 200 ml glass orange juice, 2 cups tea, whole milk, 2 sugars

Lunch
100 g chicken, 15 cm baguette with 1 tbsp mayo, 25 g packet plain
crisps, apple, 2 cups tea, whole milk, 2 sugars

Dinner
225 g grilled rump steak, 225 g jacket potato, 1 tbsp butter, 2 tbsp
poached mushrooms, 1 grilled tomato, medium bowl strawberries,
2 tbsp double cream

Snacks/drinks
2 cups coffee, whole milk and 2 sugars; 2 chocolate digestives;
2 x 175 ml glasses red wine; 1 glass water

Total calories per day: 3,048

At this pre-weight loss stage your aim is just to observe everything you eat and drink over the diary period. You are not trying to lose weight – not yet anyway. The example shows the level of detail that is required.

Food diary rules

▶ Write down everything you eat and drink, as you are eating it.

▶ Always be specific – include cooking methods, brand names, quantities (estimate as closely as you can) and varieties, e.g. 'diet drink' or 'full-fat yogurt'.

▶ Include 'hidden' ingredients such as butter in sandwiches or sugar on cereal.

Identifying calorie savings

After a few days of diary keeping it may well be that eating patterns can be seen more clearly, so that it is possible to see ways of reducing your calorie intake by swapping to lower-calorie, lower-fat foods or by reducing portion sizes. For example, from the diary it can be seen that the day's intake is high in sugar and in full-fat products, such as butter, milk and oil. The table below shows just how many calories could be saved by swapping to different varieties:

Swap this..	For this...	Calorie saving
12 tsp white sugar	12 tsp sweetener	192
300 ml whole milk	300 ml skimmed milk	90
2 tbsp double cream	2 tbsp light single cream	96
1 tbsp vegetable oil	10 sprays one-cal oil spray	125
2 x 175 ml red wine	1 x 175 ml red wine	120

Making the swaps shown above would save 623 calories in a single day – without having to make any noticeable changes to the diet. Some people will find that there are easy, daily calorie-savings they can make in their diet, whereas others may identify regular but not daily occasions – such as a weekly takeaway or a night out – where big calorie-savings can be made at a stroke. This is why it is important to keep the food diary for as long as it takes to establish a pattern.

Working out calorie needs
For a rough guide to your daily calorie needs, multiply your weight in pounds by 15 if you are moderately active; or 13 if you have a sedentary lifestyle. Using Jane as an example (see page 47), this method would estimate her total calorie needs at 2,173 compared to 2,130 for the four-step calculation.

How quickly should you lose?

Now that you know how many calories you need to maintain your weight, and how many you are currently eating each day, you can decide how much of an energy deficit you will need to set up to lose weight steadily and safely. Cutting back on food drastically – such as by sticking to a rigid 1,000 calories a day diet when your BMR is 3,000 calories – would undoubtedly lead to rapid weight loss. But it is very unlikely that you would be able to sustain it in the long term, leading to a dispiriting 'failure' and, probably, an equally rapid weight gain once you started eating normally again.

Gradual weight loss is best

Health professionals recommend that a safe and steady weight loss is about 1–2 lb (0.45–0.9 kg) a week. Slimming at this rate ensures that you will be losing fat rather than lean tissue, such as muscle, and it should be fairly easy to achieve without drastic calorie-cutting measures, so that you can stick with your plan without it feeling like a 'diet'. And, as a bonus, research shows that people who lose weight slowly are more likely to keep it off in the long run.

As it takes an energy deficit of around 3,500 calories to lose 1lb of fat, a daily saving of about 500 calories should be enough to lose 1lb a week (7 x 500). Saving 1,000 calories a day (say, from 3,000 to 2,000) could result in a 2lb weekly loss, but this depends on current intake: women should not try to lose weight on less than around 1,500 calories a day, while for men the minimum is around 1,900 calories a day.

In the first few weeks of a weight loss plan it is possible to lose more than 1lb or 2lb a week. This is because glycogen (the short-term store of surplus energy) is stored in three times its weight of water, which accounts for a lot of the initial weight loss. This can be a very motivating start to a weight-loss campaign and it may continue for longer than a week or two, especially if you have a lot of weight to lose.

There is no need for any drastic calorie cutting – or boring meals – when losing weight; healthy food can be filling and delicious.

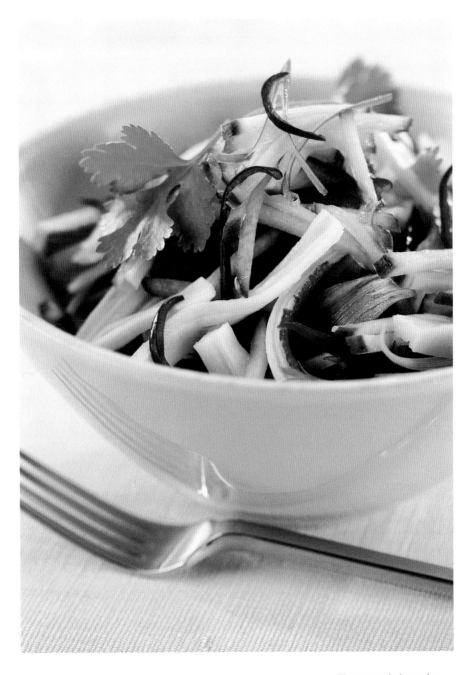

must know

Calories from alcohol
These are not stored in the body but are used immediately as energy. That sounds like good news but it's not; this is because instead the body stores calories from other sources such as fat, which tend to accumulate in fat deposits in the abdomen, and may account for the observation that many heavy drinkers are 'apple-shaped'.

Weight loss, balance and health

This chapter has looked at 'calories in and calories out', a concept which is essential to understand in order to create an energy deficit. However, it is not enough on its own to help the slimmer because it does not address the other key question: what you should eat in order to ensure that a weight loss plan is also healthy, balanced and enjoyable for you to follow.

After all, if your only aim was to lose weight by creating an energy deficit, then the diet could

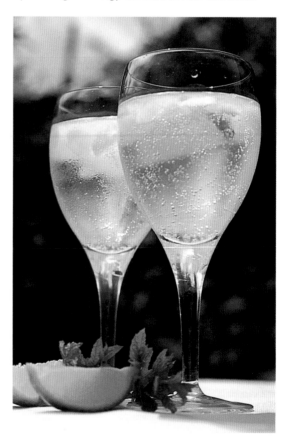

Adding lemon to a gin and tonic doesn't make it healthy! Alcoholic drinks provide 'empty calories' with little nutritional value.

consist of anything at all, as long as it saved calories. However, when you are devising an effective and personalized slimming plan, it is vital to ensure that your daily diet is healthy and balanced; that hunger is kept at bay; and that enough favourite foods are included so that the plan feels comfortable and enjoyable and you don't feel that you are missing out on meals. All of these aspects are covered in the next section.

Energy deficit

By calculating your BMR (see page 46) and your calorie intake you will build up a picture of whether your current energy balance is likely to help you maintain your weight or whether you are consistently taking in too many calories for your needs.

Adjusting both your food intake and your activity level will help to shift the balance so that you begin to lose weight; it will be important to keep a food diary (see page 48) for the first few weeks of your weight loss plan so that you can keep track of all the meals, snacks and drinks that you consume.

Once you have started this process, have done all the calculations and are sure that you are in energy deficit but you are not losing weight, then the most likely explanation is that somewhere something has been missed; it may be that daily activity has been over-estimated, or calorie intake has been under-estimated. Another week's food diary and another calculation of the 'activity factor' could reveal what has been happening.

If you still appear to be in energy deficit, you could take a short cut by looking at your daily food intake and aiming to 'save' about 500 calories a day, but make sure that you do not go below an average intake of 1,500 calories a day (women) or 1,900 calories a day (men).

want to know more?

Take it to the next level...

▶ **Recommended portion sizes** 78
▶ **Commercial calorie-controlled diets** 126
▶ **How exercise boosts weight loss** 136
▶ **Calories used in different activities** 150

Other sources
▶ **See page 180 for your Personal Record Planner of diet and fitness progress.**
▶ **Ask if your gym has a machine that quickly calculates your BMR by testing your breath.**
▶ **Look out for websites that allow you to fill in an online diary and predict how long it will take you to reach your target weight.**
▶ **If you're uncertain about working on your own calorie-controlled diet, consult a qualified nutritionist or dietitian.**
▶ **Follow the calorie-controlled menu plans in women's magazines or slimming magazines to get you started or for extra inspiration.**

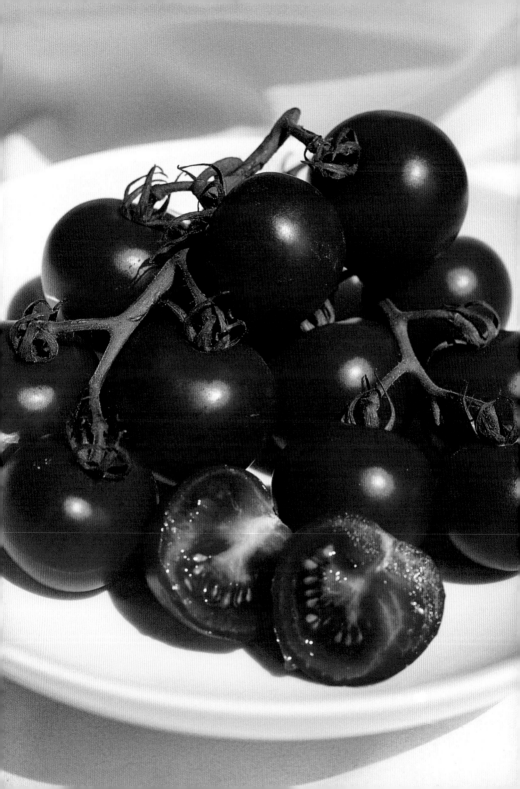

5 Healthy eating for slimmers

As losing weight is about improving health as well as looking and feeling confident, it makes sense to ensure that any weight loss plan is as healthy as possible. Knowing how to create filling, tasty menus that contain a wide range of nutrients, but without piling on the calories or fat, is the key to finding a way of eating that is easy to follow, enjoyable and effective in managing your weight.

Getting the balance right

A key message from health professionals is that there is no such thing as healthy or unhealthy foods – only healthy or unhealthy diets. To lose weight in a healthy way, it is especially important to know how to get the balance right.

Super groups

Eating in a healthy way is about getting the right combination of nutrients, or all the compounds the body needs to function efficiently. There are two different and distinct groups of nutrients in foods: macronutrients, which are protein, carbohydrates, fats and water; and micronutrients, which are vitamins and minerals.

The body needs different amounts of nutrients to function healthily, such as quite large quantities of carbohydrate, and tiny amounts of vitamins and minerals. Getting the balance wrong can have all sorts of negative consequences for health, which range from feeling generally 'under par' to serious conditions such as anaemia (not enough iron) or osteoporosis (not enough calcium).

Most foods are a mixture of nutrients: dairy products, for instance, contain protein, fats, micronutrients and water, while rice contains carbohydrate, protein, fat, micronutrients and water.

Balance of Good Health

Having to keep track of the nutrients in every food would make it very difficult to devise a balanced diet, and would turn mealtimes into a chemistry lesson instead of an enjoyable event. So when

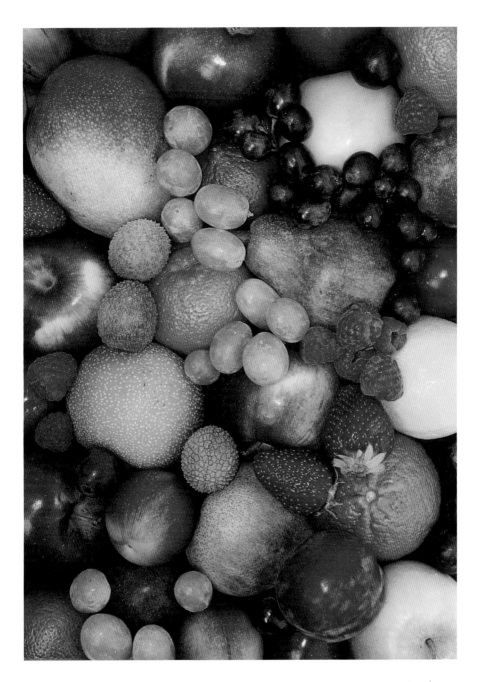

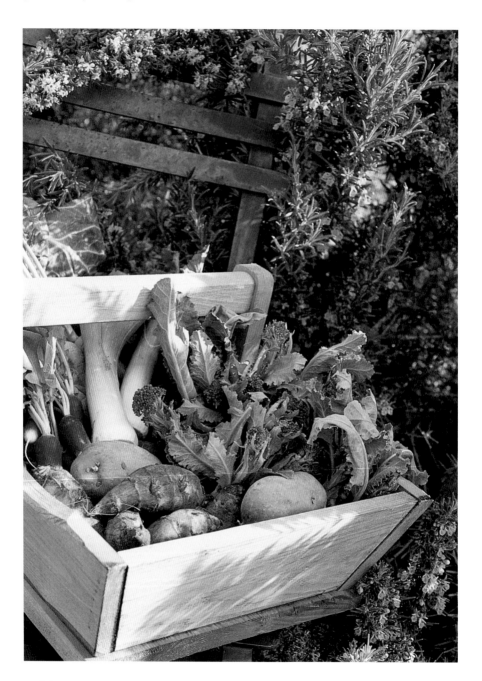

nutritionists talk about 'food groups' they are referring to the types of everyday foods that are needed to make up a healthy diet. The Government's Food Standards Agency describes the ideal combination of food groups in terms of the 'Balance of Good Health' plate. These groups are as follows:

- Fruit and vegetables
- Bread, other cereals and potatoes
- Milk and dairy foods
- Meat, fish and alternatives
- Foods containing fats and sugars.

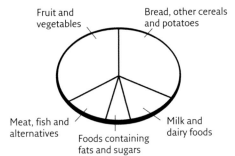

There is no need to give up any of the above food groups in order to have a healthy diet – not even sugary and fatty foods; the key to healthy eating is to bear in mind the proportions.

Food groups for slimmers

We have already seen that in order to lose weight, the most important factor is to create an energy deficit (see page 45) so that more calories are expended in energy than are consumed as foods. However, it is essential that when you are cutting down on calories, the overall balance of your diet remains healthy. The Balance of Good Health is a useful blueprint for people who want to lose weight as well as for people who want to maintain a healthy weight, and the good news for slimmers is that, as long as the overall energy intake is controlled, they, too, can and should enjoy foods from all the food groups.

Nutritionists advise against weight-loss diets that cut out one or more major food groups, partly because they can be monotonous and harder to stick to, but also because avoiding any food group could risk missing out on valuable nutrients. This is even true of the 'fatty and sugary foods' group, as some fats are essential for good health.

A treasure trove of health: eating plenty of fresh seasonal vegetables ensures that you are benefiting from all the nutrients that they contain.

Reducing salt
Slimmers can cut down on salt and calories by cooking fresh food instead of relying just on convenience foods: flavouring meals with pepper and herbs instead of salt; and buying canned fish and vegetables in water rather than brine or oil.

Fruit and vegetables for health

Fruit and vegetables are the biggest single food group in the Balance of Good Health guidelines for a healthy diet (see page 59). Adults are recommended to eat at least five 80 g portions of fruit and vegetables a day – a total of 400 g or more – although currently only around four out of 10 people in the UK manage to follow these guidelines.

Health benefits

Experts believe that eating at least the recommended amount of fruit and vegetables each day could reduce the risk of dying from diseases such as cancer, heart disease and stroke by up to 20 per cent. This is thought to be the second most important cancer prevention strategy after giving up smoking.

Research has also shown that each increase of one portion of fruit and vegetables a day lowers the risk of developing coronary heart disease by four per cent and the risk of stroke by six per cent.

Fruity facts

One 150 ml glass of fruit juice or 150 ml fruit smoothie counts as one fruit portion, but for health purposes can only be counted once a day; canned and dried fruit also count. However, as the table below shows, processed fruit in all its forms is usually higher in energy density than fresh, which means that it has more calories weight for weight and is less filling, so it is not always the best choice for slimmers.

Fruit serving	Calories
100 g white grapes	12
112 g/4 oz medium apple	53
28 g/1 oz dried apple slices	67
28 g/1 oz raisins/sultanas	82
200 ml glass grape juice	92
200 ml glass apple juice	95
200 ml apple & grape smoothie	100

Not all fruit are low in calories: avocados can be up to 80 per cent fat – although it is the more healthy monounsaturated kind of fat.

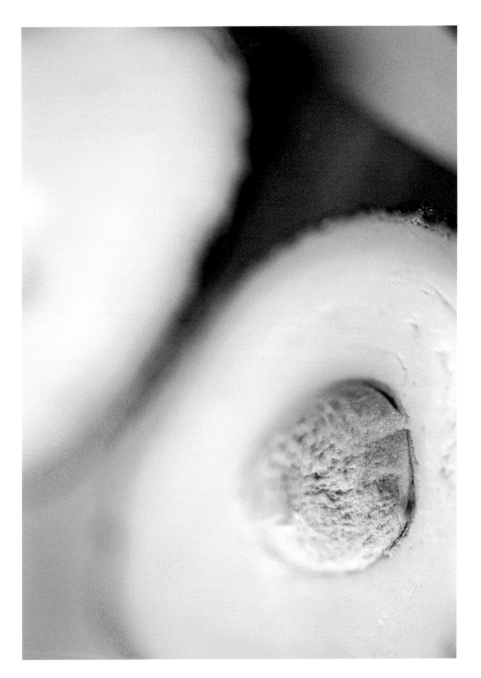

must know

Eat a 'rainbow'
Many of the valuable plant compounds in fruit and vegetables are also the ones that give them their colour, such as the red pigment lycopene in tomatoes, which has anti-cancer properties. The skin of purple grapes contains flavonoids – antioxidants that protect body cells – and bright vegetables like peppers are rich in vitamin C. However, as all fruit and vegetables are good for health, it is better to stick to favourite kinds rather than not eat any at all.

The other health benefits of eating plenty of fruit and vegetables include delaying the development of cataracts, lowering blood pressure, helping to manage diabetes, improving bowel function and reducing the symptoms of asthma.

While five portions a day is recommended as the level for good health, it is still worth bearing in mind that this is a minimum and is partly based on what is thought to be acceptable. In some other countries, including the United States, the guideline is nine portions a day.

Fruit and vegetables are especially beneficial to our health because of the wide range of compounds that they contain. These include vitamins and minerals as well as complex plant components – phytochemicals – which, among other valuable functions, play an essential 'antioxidant' role in

Fruit can truly claim to be a 'superfood' for anyone who is trying to lose weight.

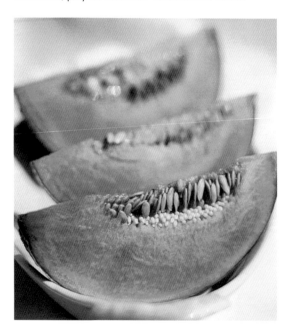

preventing damage and disease to cells. It is believed that these compounds work most efficiently when taken in conjunction with each other; eating them on their own, in the form of food supplements, does not have the same beneficial effects and can occasionally even do more harm than good.

Superfoods for slimmers

Eating more fruit and vegetables is one of the most common changes that successful slimmers make to their diet, and many report that it is the single most important change they make. This is because fruit and vegetables can truly claim to be 'superfoods' for anyone who is trying to lose weight.

The main reason for this is that most fruit and vegetables are bulky and watery, which means that they are low in energy density – in other words, they

Vegetables from the onion family contain allicin, a phytochemical with numerous health benefits.

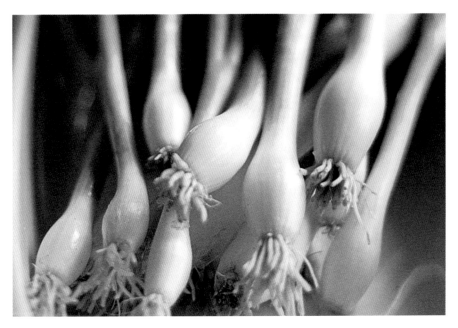

must know

Excess salt
Most people in the UK eat too much salt; the recommended level for adults is 6 g (about a teaspoon) a day, and on average we eat 9.5 g a day, most of it in processed food such as ready meals, soups and sauces. Excess salt is bad for health, as it raises blood pressure which, in turn, increases the risk of heart disease and stroke. This is especially bad news for slimmers, as overweight people are already likely to be at risk of high blood pressure. Too much salt can also encourage fluid retention and can deplete the body of calcium, which protects bones and plays a part in the metabolism of fat.

can provide a large and filling volume of food for relatively few calories. Many fruit and vegetables are also high in fibre, which is filling and helps maintain a feeling of fullness. In addition, many have a low glycaemic index (GI) rating, and this means that they release energy slowly into the bloodstream, which can help reduce the need to snack between meals.

People who eat lots of fruit and vegetables also tend to eat fewer fatty and sugary foods, which is a big help in controlling overall calorie intake and creating the energy deficit necessary for losing weight. For all these reasons, a healthy eating plan for weight loss can include generous amounts of most fruit and vegetables, with five portions a day as the minimum, as long as no fat or sugar is added in cooking or serving. For the 80 g portion size of a number of different fruit and vegetables, see page 56.

Key points
These guidelines will help you to enjoy fruit and vegetables as part of a weight loss diet:
▶ Fresh, frozen or canned fruit and vegetables are all good for health; for weight loss, choose varieties with no added fat or sugar (such as fruit syrup).
▶ Fruit and vegetable juices and dried fruit are full of nutrients but energy-dense, so count the calories.
▶ Start a meal with a salad or vegetable soup; studies show that slimmers who do this eat fewer calories overall than those who have just a main course.

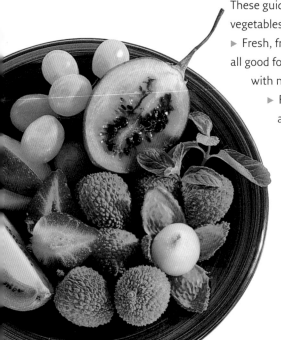

Cut calories at a stroke by swapping sugary snacks for a piece of fruit.

Bread, cereals and potatoes

These account for just under a third of the 'Balance of Good Health' plate (see page 59). This second-largest group is important as it features foods that are rich in starchy carbohydrates, including potatoes which, despite being a vegetable, appear in this group because they are counted as a starchy food. Starchy carbohydrates are an essential part of our diet because they provide energy: they are broken down by digestion to produce glucose, which is stored in the liver and muscles or circulated in the bloodstream, then used for our immediate energy needs.

Adding fresh fruit to a bowl of breakfast cereal is a good first step to five-a-day.

Starchy carbohydrates, especially whole-grain sources, such as wholemeal bread and pasta, brown rice and bran cereals, are also high in dietary fibre, which is important for satisfying the appetite and keeping the digestive system working efficiently.

Some carbohydrate-rich foods, such as porridge oats, have a low glycaemic index (GI) rating, which means that they release glucose slowly into the bloodstream, keeping blood sugar levels stable and helping to keep the appetite satisfied for longer. People with diabetes are usually advised to eat plenty of starchy, high-fibre foods in order to help regulate their blood sugar. Micronutrients in starchy carbohydrate foods include some calcium, iron and B vitamins; many common brands of bread and breakfast cereals are also fortified with these nutrients.

Versatile eating

There is such a rich variety of bread, cereals and grains that it is possible to create thousands of meals by exploring different types: for instance, try couscous instead of pasta with tomato sauce or roasted vegetables; noodles instead of rice with Chinese dishes; or sweet potato instead of standard potato as a pie topping.

must know

Wheat allergies
People who are allergic to wheat can still enjoy foods from the bread and cereals group, such as rye, oats and rice.

Carbohydrates for slimmers

The fact that bread, cereals and potatoes are considered to be such a key part of a healthy diet may be surprising to slimmers who have been led to believe that starchy foods, especially bread and potatoes, are 'fattening'. In fact, carbohydrates are relatively low in calories weight for weight, with just four calories per gram; this makes them good value in terms of 'energy density' as they are bulky, filling and take time to eat – all good news for slimmers.

That said, starchy foods are the perfect partners for high-calorie foods, such as fats and sugars. Pasta with creamy sauce, jacket potatoes with butter and sugar-coated breakfast cereals all add hundreds of calories to starchy foods and make them easier to eat, which means it's not difficult to overeat them without noticing. Bread in particular can be a 'trigger food' for some slimmers, who find it hard to control their portions.

Key points

Here are some useful guidelines to help you to enjoy bread, cereals and potatoes when you are on a weight loss diet:
► Choose high-fibre, whole-grain, brown or wholemeal versions wherever possible.
► If adding fat when cooking or serving food, keep it to a minimum and count the calories.
► Look out for hidden fats and sugars in carbohydrate-rich foods, such as bread made with oil, or sugary breakfast cereals.
► Eat jacket potatoes and boiled new potatoes in their skins to maximize vitamin C, filling power and fibre.

Milk and dairy foods for health

Milk and all the products that are derived from it – cheese, yogurt, fromage frais and many more – are the third biggest group in the Balance of Good Health (see page 59), making up just over a sixth of the total. Dairy produce is a good source of protein, which is essential for growth and maintenance of the body's tissues. It is also rich in calcium, a mineral which is vital to build and maintain strong bones and teeth, especially in women and young people, and also has many other valuable functions to fulfil in the body. In addition to being a good source of calcium, dairy produce also provides vitamins B12, A and D.

However, full-fat dairy produce is energy-dense and can be eaten very quickly, so it is easy to pile on the fat and calories without even noticing. The fat that it contains is also of the saturated variety, which may contribute to a higher risk of developing heart disease. The Balance of Good Health recommendation is to have only moderate amounts of dairy produce and to choose lower-fat varieties where possible.

must know

Sensitivities and allergies
People who are sensitive to cow's milk can try products made from goat's milk or sheep's milk; those who are allergic to all dairy products can choose from milk and yogurts made from calcium-enriched soya milk or rice milk.

Facing the fats

The table below shows the amount of fat and calories in 100 g of a range of cheeses, from full-fat Cheddar to very low-fat fromage frais. Huge savings in fat and calories can be made by switching from hard to soft cheeses and from full-fat to reduced-fat versions.

Cheese type	Fat per 100 g	Calories per 100 g
Cream cheese	47.4	439
Cheddar	34.4	412
Processed cheese	27	330
Soft full-fat cheese	31	313
Camembert	23.7	297
Full-fat cheese spread	22.8	276
Reduced-fat Cheddar	15	261
Soft medium-fat cheese	14.5	179
Plain fromage frais	7.1	113
Plain cottage cheese	3.9	98
Reduced-fat cottage cheese	1.4	78
Very low fat fromage frais	0.2	58

Milk and dairy foods for slimmers

Now that there are so many low-fat versions of milk and dairy products available, slimmers need never miss out on the nutrients provided by this food group: skimmed milk, for example, is higher in calcium than full-fat milk. Not all low-fat products are low in calories, as sugars may be added to replace fats in desserts, for instance, but plain low-fat versions can provide plenty of creamy taste without all the calories and saturated fat.

Recent research shows that eating calcium-rich, low-fat dairy products may be especially beneficial for slimmers because calcium appears to play a role in helping fat metabolize more efficiently; in trials, people who ate low-fat yogurt as part of a weight loss diet did better than those who did not. The same effect was not seen when calcium was taken on its own, as a supplement. Like bread, cheese can be an eating trigger for some slimmers who find it hard to resist; as it is calorie-dense and easy to eat, watching portion sizes is important.

Key points

Here are some helpful guidelines for enjoying milk and dairy foods as part of a weight loss diet:

▶ Try different varieties of reduced-fat cheese and dairy products to find the ones that taste best.

▶ Having a daily allowance for milk in drinks and on cereals can help control overall calorie intake.

▶ Read the labels on 'healthy' yogurt drinks and smoothies, which can be high in calories and sugar.

▶ Allow for 600 ml (1 pint) of skimmed milk or the equivalent in low-fat dairy products each day to ensure sufficient calcium intake.

▶ Make hard cheese go further by grating rather than slicing, or making it into sauce with skimmed milk.

▶ Look out for opportunities to cut down on excess dairy fat – for instance, by doing without spread in sandwiches or not piling butter on vegetables.

Meat, fish and proteins for health

Meat, fish and other sources of protein are the smallest of the four main food groups in the Balance of Good Health (see page 59), accounting for just under one-sixth of the foods we eat.

Lean meat and fish are the principal sources of protein in the diet; protein is also found in eggs and dairy produce. It is an essential component of the diet because when it is digested it produces amino acids, which are the building blocks of cells and tissues; carbohydrates and fats cannot produce amino acids. Red meat is a good source of iron, in a form which is more easily available to the body than iron from other sources, such as vegetables. Fatty meat though can be higher in calories and also in

Eggs pack plenty of protein, but if you have high cholesterol aim to eat no more than three a week.

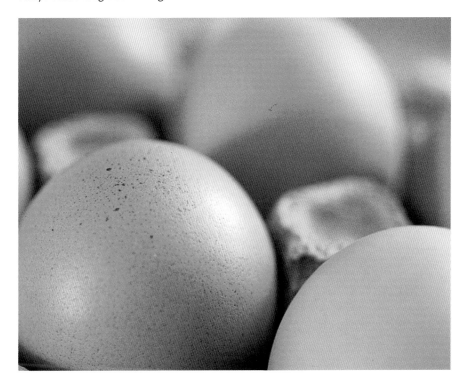

saturated fat. Protein-rich foods also provide other important nutrients such as B vitamins, zinc and magnesium.

Oily fish, such as mackerel, sardines and salmon, are a good source of omega 3 essential fatty acids, which are beneficial to heart health because they can help reduce the levels of LDL cholesterol in the blood, and may also protect against strokes.

Meat, fish and proteins for slimmers

Like carbohydrates, proteins are also low in energy density, with four calories per gram. Protein is very satiating, which means it is a filling food and therefore a good choice for slimmers. Some people find that protein-rich foods, such as a lean steak or piece of fresh tuna, are more satisfying than carbohydrates and make a filling, tasty meal with plenty of green vegetables instead of potatoes or bread. Lean cuts of meat, game and offal are low in fat, and so is fish, with the exception of oily fish, which is relatively high in fat and calories. However, it is important to eat this once a week because it contains omega 3 essential fatty acids. Nuts and seeds, while rich in many vitamins, minerals and beneficial plant compounds, are high in calories; a 50 g bag of salted peanuts, for instance, has around 300 calories and 40 g fat and is very quick to eat.

Key points

In order to enjoy meat, fish and protein foods in a weight loss diet, follow these simple guidelines:

▶ Remove all visible fat from meat and poultry before cooking, including poultry skin.

▶ Choose lower-fat versions of processed meats, such as sausages, bacon and burgers, and do not eat these every day.

▶ Avoid meat and fish dishes that are deep-fried, coated in breadcrumbs or in creamy sauces.

▶ Experiment with no-fat cooking methods for meat and fish, such as braising, baking, grilling, poaching, barbecuing and steaming.

▶ Choose the leanest cuts of meat, including extra-lean mince.

Fatty and sugary foods for health

Foods containing fat and those containing sugar are the smallest group in the Balance of Good Health (see page 59), accounting for under 10 per cent of the total food intake. On many people's plates, however, they account for far more than this; on average, people in the UK eat 7.2 kg of crisps and 24 kg of sugar each every year. Retail surveys also show that we buy an average of 372 snacks each per year, most of them high in fat, sugar or both.

Many of the high-fat, high-sugar foods that we eat are processed foods, ranging from fast foods and pastries, cakes and buns, to sweets, chocolates, drinks, savoury snacks, sauces and dressings.

Sweet tooth? Count 16 calories for every teaspoon of sugar.

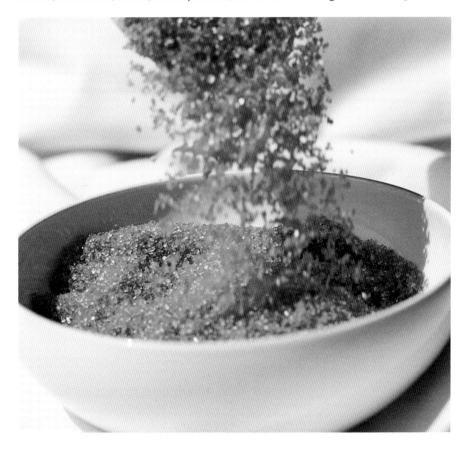

must know

Get the balance right
To eat healthily, it is not essential to have a carefully-balanced plate at every meal, but you should be aware of the importance of getting the balance right over the course of a day or a week.

All high-fat, high-sugar foods provide energy in the form of simple or refined carbohydrates, but as they are nearly always calorie-dense, appetizing and quick to eat, it is easy to see why they are routinely blamed for our growing weight problem. The fat in processed foods is often saturated animal fat, which is associated with high blood cholesterol, which can clog arteries. Some processed foods are made with hydrogenated vegetable fats, which may sound healthy but are in fact implicated in the development of heart disease. Eating lots of high-fat, high-sugar foods also makes it less likely that people will eat healthier foods such as fruit, vegetables and complex carbohydrates.

We need some fat

However, some fat is essential in the diet. Its functions include helping to keep the immune system and reproductive system running smoothly and it contains the fat-soluble vitamins A, D, E and K. Plant oils contain monounsaturated or polyunsaturated fats, which contain no cholesterol and have compounds that may benefit heart health. Sugar has no nutritional value other than as a readily-available source of energy.

Fatty and sugary foods for slimmers

Along with eating more fruit and vegetables, cutting right down on fatty and sugary foods is the other big change that slimmers say contributes to successful weight loss. Fats are the most calorie-dense of all the food groups: each gram of fat provides nine calories, which is why cutting down on fat is one of the easiest ways of all to reduce our overall energy intake. As a carbohydrate, sugar has four calories per gram but the danger for slimmers is that it is very easy to add large quantities of calories to food in the form of sugar without adding any volume at all – think of sugar stirred into tea or sprinkled onto cereal.

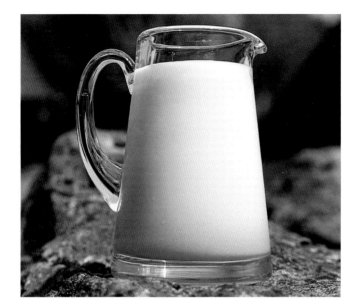

Skimmed milk has more calcium, less fat and fewer calories than whole milk.

Including a few sugary sweets in the diet may not necessarily be bad news; studies have found that slimmers who ate a daily sugar-rich snack of boiled sweets or fudge as part of a weight-loss diet did better than those who did not. Eating a little more sugar may result in eating less fat, and having sweets may reduce any cravings for sugar between meals, but, as ever, it is the overall calorie intake that matters.

Key points

Here are some useful guidelines for enjoying fatty and sugary foods in a weight loss diet:

▶ Replace sugar in hot drinks with sweetener, if liked, or try unsweetened drinks such as fruit or herbal teas.

▶ Use fat sparingly to add flavour to meals, e.g. a little oil to brush over roasted vegetables or make a low-fat salad dressing.

▶ Keep proportions in mind when choosing high-fat dishes such as pizza or curry; balance out a small portion by piling the plate with salad, boiled rice or vegetables.

Key micronutrients at a glance

The information below is based on advice from the Food Standards Agency's website, which has a lot more detail on a wide range of nutrients. Generally, we should be able to get all the vitamins and minerals we need from food, as long as we eat a balanced diet. Overdosing on certain vitamins, such as vitamin A, can be harmful: pregnant women in particular should avoid large amounts. If you are worried that your diet may be vitamin-deficient or need advice on supplements, ask your GP.

Micronutrient	Good sources	Function
Vitamin A (retinol)	Dairy produce; liver	Maintains health of skin and tissues; immune function; night vision.
Vitamin B6 (pyridoxine)	Meat, fish, cereals	Energy metabolism; helps form haemoglobin.
Vitamin B12	Meat, dairy produce	Formation of blood cells and nerve fibres.
Carotenes	Fruit and vegetables	Antioxidant; help vitamin A to function.
Vitamin C (ascorbic acid)	Fruit and vegetables	Antioxidant; helps protect cells from damage.
Vitamin D	Oily fish, liver, eggs	Helps regulate minerals that are essential for healthy teeth and bones.
Vitamin E	Plant oils, nuts, seeds, wheatgerm	Antioxidant; helps protect cells from damage.
Vitamin K	Green leafy vegetables, vegetable oils, cereals	Wound healing, helps build strong bones.
Calcium (mineral)	Dairy products; green leafy vegetables, oily fish	Essential for healthy teeth and bones; helps metabolism; cell structure.
Iron (mineral)	Meat, fish and proteins, fortified bread and cereals, dark green vegetables.	Essential for forming haemoglobin (transports oxygen in the blood)
Magnesium (mineral)	Meat, fish and proteins	Bone development; nerve and muscle function; enzyme function.
Potassium (mineral)	Fruit and vegetables; meat	Regulates fluids in the body; may help regulate blood pressure.
Zinc (trace element)	Meat, fish and proteins	Tissue growth; immune function; wound healing.

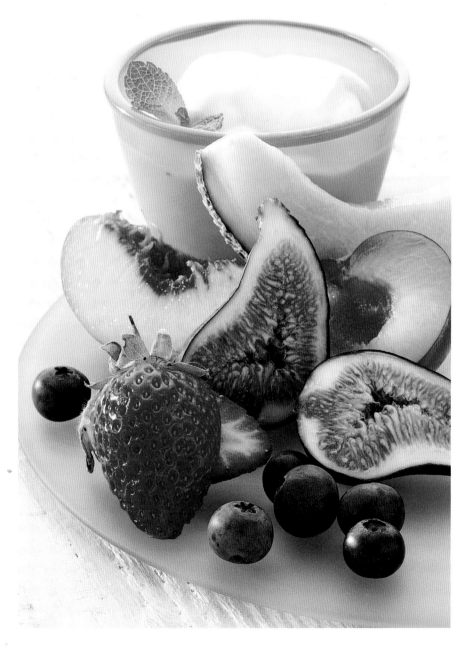

Alcohol
Moderate amounts, e.g. one or
two small glasses of red wine or a
pint of beer a day, may be mildly
beneficial to health, but the
calories in alcohol are 'empty',
supplying virtually no nutritional
value. Count around 100 calories
for a glass of wine, 300 ml beer or
lager or a double measure of
spirits. Mixed drinks (cocktails
and alcopops) are higher still, as
are extra-strong lagers and beers.
Alcohol is bad news in other ways:
it is a depressant and not good
for self-esteem; it boosts appetite
for salty foods and snacks, and
weakens self-control. Cutting
down on alcohol is an easy way
to reduce calorie intake without
missing out on nutrients.

Fibre for health

Dietary fibre comes in two forms: insoluble and
soluble. As the name suggests, insoluble fibre does
not dissolve in the digestive tract; it passes straight
through, providing bulk which helps food and waste
move more efficiently through the system and
preventing bowel problems such as constipation.
Soluble fibre dissolves in the digestive tract and has
a different function; it can help to reduce cholesterol
in the bloodstream and so benefit heart health.
Good sources of insoluble fibre are foods made with
wheat bran, such as bran cereals, wholegrain bread
and wholemeal pasta; vegetables and pulses.
Soluble fibre is found in non-wheat cereals such
as oats, barley and rye, and in fruit.

There are many good reasons why slimmers
should include plenty of high-fibre foods in the diet.
High-fibre foods tend to be slow to eat and chew, so
they contribute to a feeling of fullness. They are low
in energy density, so they provide volume without
a large quantity of calories, and they are slow to pass through
the digestive system, so the feeling of fullness persists, helping
to prevent 'snack attacks'. Slimmers who start eating a lot more
fibre may find they feel bloated or even show a weight gain
at first: this is likely to be a short-term effect as fibre absorbs
water. Drinking plenty of liquids will help to get the system
running smoothly again and assuming the overall energy intake
is reduced, weight loss will result in time.

Be smart with servings

Knowing the kinds of foods to eat when slimming is one thing;
knowing how much to eat of everything is another. Unless they
are trying to lose weight, most people don't bother weighing and
measuring food and drinks. The portion sizes of many pre-packaged

foods have increased, especially sweets, snacks, fast food takeaways and restaurant meals. As a result, it is easy to lose sight of what standard servings look like in the overall balance of a healthy diet.

Weighing and measuring

Some weighing and measuring is inevitable when getting to grips with serving sizes and reducing overall energy intake. It only takes a small daily surplus of calories to create a weight problem over time; checking portion sizes and keeping a food diary are key skills in achieving slimming success. Not every mouthful has to be monitored for life; with practice, it gets easier to estimate portion sizes of different foods and get used to the proportions of meals that satisfy the appetite without sending the calorie-count soaring.

Portions in proportion: there is room for all the food groups - plus a dessert - in a balanced meal.

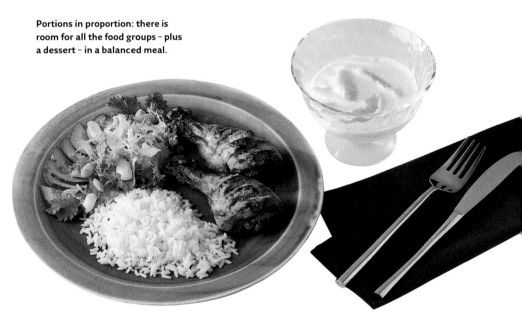

How many servings?

When deciding on the number of servings of each food group to eat at each meal, it is important to take some key factors into account:

Overall Balance of Good Health

Choose the largest number of servings from the Bread, Cereals and Potatoes (see page 65) and Fruit and Vegetables groups (see page 60), with fewer servings of protein-rich foods and dairy produce, and fatty and sugary foods kept to a minimum.

Overall calorie intake

The total number of calories eaten each day will vary; people with a lot of weight to lose or who are very active will need more calories than inactive people who only want to lose a few pounds. The more calories needed, the more servings can be chosen, but the balance

---

Typical serving sizes

The British Dietetic Association (BDA) recommends these typical single serving sizes of foods from the major food groups. Choose the number of servings from each group that suits you each day.

Bread, cereals and potatoes	Meat, fish and proteins	Milk and dairy foods	Fats and oils
1 slice of bread or toast	60–90 g (2–3 oz) cooked lean meat, poultry or oily fish	200 ml glass of milk	1 tsp butter, margarine, oil, mayonnaise or double cream
2 crispbreads	2 thin slices lean ham or bacon	1 small pot of yogurt or fromage frais	
3 tbsp breakfast cereals		1 small matchbox size of hard cheese	2 tsp reduced-fat spread or salad dressing
2 egg-sized potatoes	150 g (5 oz) cooked white fish or canned tuna	90 g (3 oz) cottage cheese	
2 heaped tbsp boiled rice		60 g (2 oz) low-fat soft cheese	
3 heaped tbsp boiled pasta	2 eggs		
Half a fruit or plain scone	5 tbsp baked beans		
	4 tbsp peas or pulses		
	120 g (4 oz) of soya or tofu		

---

on the plate, or over the day's eating, from the different food groups should always remain roughly the same.

Appetite satisfaction

When choosing what to eat it is important to ensure that hunger pangs are not a problem and that the daily calorie allowance does not run out through the day. This is more likely to happen if too many servings of calorie-dense foods and not enough servings of fruit, vegetables and starchy foods are chosen. Having servings of starchy foods at every meal will help keep blood sugar levels stable and satisfy the appetite.

Personal preference

Many slimmers worry that they will have to eat many foods that they do not like when they start a diet. However, this is not true; it is possible to lose weight healthily without eating, say, cottage

Eating out need not be off the menu just because you are slimming.

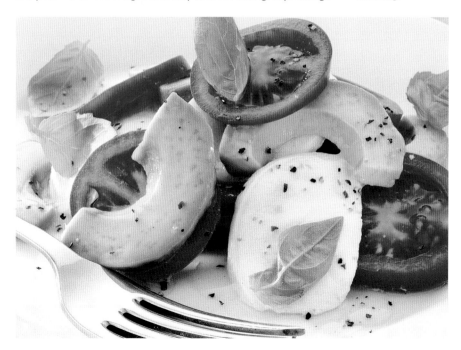

Eating out

These days many people in the UK eat out more often than they do at home – potentially a recipe for ruining any weight loss plan as calories and fat can pile up very quickly. The table below lists some helpful and not-so-helpful choices for slimmers at popular types of restaurant.

Restaurant	Yes please	No thank you
Chinese	Clear soup; stir fried vegetables; steamed or grilled meat or fish; dishes in light sauce (black bean or oyster); boiled rice	Sweet & sour dishes; egg fried rice; prawn toasts; banana fritters
French	Vegetable soup; seafood salad; grilled meat, fish or poultry; fresh fruit salad; sorbet	Pâté; cream sauces; butter; dauphinois potatoes; profiteroles; gâteaux
Greek	Egg and lemon soup; stuffed vine leaves; hummus; pitta bread; grilled kebabs; steak; fresh tuna; figs with yogurt	Taramasalata; moussaka; stifado; kleftiko; baklava
Indian	Tandoori dishes; vegetable curry; dhal; boiled rice; chapatti; 'dry' meat curry	Creamy curry sauces; pilau rice; stuffed naan bread; deep-fried vegetables.
Italian	Parma ham with melon; pasta with tomato, vegetable or seafood sauce; grilled meat or fish with vegetables; sorbet or fresh fruit salad	Deep-fried mushrooms; creamy pasta sauces; risotto; gâteaux; tiramisu
Thai	Hot & sour soup; steamed fish; grilled meat; boiled rice; stir-fry vegetables; tropical fruit	Deep-fried starters; coconut milk curries; fried rice; satay sauce
Pub	Carvery roast (new potatoes); mixed grill (no chips); vegetable chilli with rice; jacket potato; lean meat and salad; ice cream, strawberries	Creamy bakes; bangers and mash; scampi; pastry pies; sponge puddings; cheesecake
Coffee shop	'Skinny' or black coffee; fruit or herb tea; fruit juice; plain scone; soup; wholemeal roll; pitta.	Super-size servings; filled baguettes; croissants; pastries.
Burger bar	Standard burger or chicken burger (extra salad, hold the mayo), small portion fries	Extra-large portions; extra cheese; mayonnaise; doughnuts; full-sugar drinks
Fish & chip shop	Fish (remove batter); small portion chips; mushy peas or baked beans; chicken kebab and salad; chilli relish	Battered sausages; fishcakes; pies; mayonnaise; fruit fritters
Sandwich bar	Wholemeal bread (no spread); lean meat; poultry or tuna filling; extra salad; jacket potato with tuna, beans or prawns; fresh fruit	Butter; fillings with mayonnaise; speciality bread (e.g. ciabatta); full-fat cheese; quiche; pastries

cheese, salads or Brussels sprouts – experiment to find foods from each group that taste good. It is also true that any weight loss plan is much easier to stick to if it includes an individual's favourite foods. A serving or two of fatty or sugary foods, such as a small chocolate bar or packet of crisps, a small glass of wine or a slice of cake, can easily be fitted into a calorie-controlled day and can make all the difference between success and failure.

Be energy aware

We have already seen how different food groups vary in energy density, i.e. the number of calories they have, weight for weight. Energy-dense foods, such as cream or chocolate, pack a lot of calories into a small volume and can be eaten very quickly, compared to low energy-dense foods, such as apples or pasta.

It is clear to see how knowing about energy density can benefit slimmers: low energy-dense foods tend to be bulky, watery or both, so that they provide appetite-satisfying volume without huge numbers of calories. They also tend to be low in fat and high in fibre, making them good for health as well as for weight loss. Foods that are low in energy density include fruit and vegetables, starchy foods including potatoes and pulses, lean meat, white fish, and low-fat dairy produce. As long as other foods are measured, it is still possible to eat unlimited amounts of these foods and still lose weight.

The concept of low energy-density diets for weight loss has recently attracted renewed interest; the prestigious Mayo Clinic in the United States has devised its own version, whereas in the UK, Slimming World pioneered the idea with Food Optimising and was followed in 2005 by Weight Watchers with its No Count plan.

want to know more?

Take it to the next level...

▶ **Keeping a food diary** 48
▶ **How to create an energy deficit** 50
▶ **Low-fat diets** 94
▶ **High-fibre diets** 96
▶ **Glycaemic index (GI)** 98

Other sources
▶ **Buy a reference book listing calorie and fat values of basic and branded foods.**
▶ **Invest in good-quality kitchen scales, a measuring jug and spoons for checking serving sizes.**
▶ **Try kitchen shops for healthy-eating gadgets such as grills, slow cookers, steamers, non-stick pans, blenders and woks.**
▶ **Buy dried or fresh herbs, spices, pepper, garlic and chilli to add flavour to savoury meals instead of salt.**
▶ **Look in food magazines and cookery books for enticing low-fat, low-calorie recipes.**
▶ **For more on salt and health, see: www.salt.gov.uk**
▶ **For more on The Balance of Good Health, see: www.nutrition.org.uk**

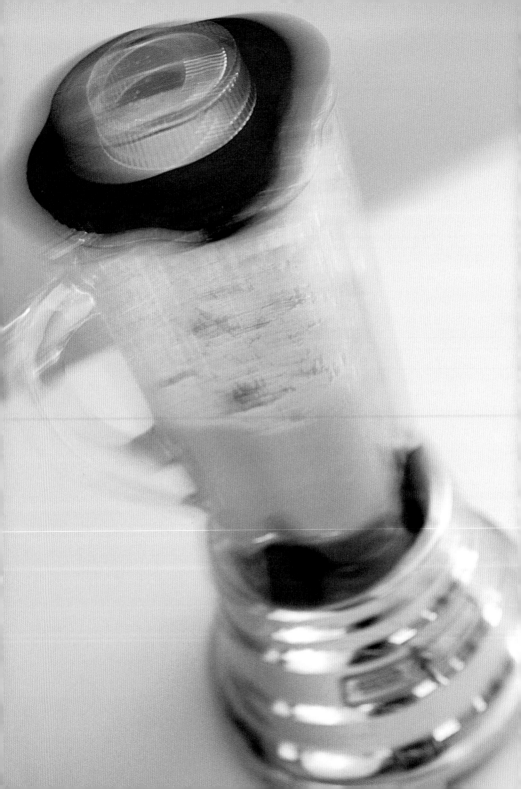

6 Choosing a weight loss method

With so many claims and counter-claims about the healthiest and most effective ways to lose weight, it can be difficult to know which method to choose. This section includes a concise profile of over 30 different diet plans and other aids to slimming, together with a simple guide to how to assess their claims, and some useful information on where to seek out the best professional advice on weight loss.

Where to get good advice

Just as there are many different types of weight loss diets, there are also many sources of personal help available. Here is some advice on where and how to seek it.

Options and services

Most people would probably think of their GP as the first port of call with any health-related issue, and many primary care teams are responding to the growing obesity problem by increasing the range of options they have to offer.

Clinical and lifestyle services

These could include 'clinical' services, such as being referred to a dietitian within the practice or at a hospital, or to a specialist hospital obesity clinic, clinical psychologist or counsellor. Services that take a more 'lifestyle' approach could include referral 'on prescription' to a local fitness centre or responsible slimming club, an invitation to join a slimming group held at the practice, or the recommendation of a qualified complementary therapist, such as an acupuncturist or hypnotherapist.

Because of demands on the NHS's time and budgets, clinical services are likely to be reserved for people with severe, longstanding weight problems which are causing weight-related illnesses or 'co-morbidities'. For the majority of overweight people who need regular support and advice, lifestyle approaches are likely to become much more widespread in the future. In its 2005 White Paper on public health, for example, the British Government set out plans for personal health advisers to work in the community – they would not necessarily be medically qualified but would be trained to offer support on a range of different areas including weight and fitness.

Weight management professionals working in the NHS are likely to be either dietitians, who have a state registration in dietetics (SRD) and are members of the British Dietetic Association (BDA), or registered nutritionists (RNutr), who are qualified members of the Nutrition Society.

must know

Pregnant women
Women who are pregnant or trying to conceive and wish to lose weight should always ask their doctor's advice first.

Complementary therapists

The only complementary therapists who are subject to statutory regulation are osteopaths and chiropractors. Terms such as 'nutritionist', 'therapist', 'practitioner' or 'coach' can be used by advisers without specific qualifications, and the qualifications they do have may not be recognized by mainstream medicine. The British Association for Nutritional Therapy (BANT), which takes a complementary approach to weight management, is working to have its standards recognized by the NHS and the Department of Health; other organizations prefer to operate outside the mainstream.

Healthy eating will be much easier if you like the foods that are on offer.

Some weight loss advisers do not offer diet plans but are lifestyle coaches, aiming to help clients boost their motivation and achieve their goals, usually based on a weekly one-to-one consultation. Most practitioners working outside the NHS do not require a GP referral; it is important to assess carefully in advance what they will charge for advice, whether you will be required to buy any other products (such as supplements) and whether you feel that what they have to offer seems to suit what you need.

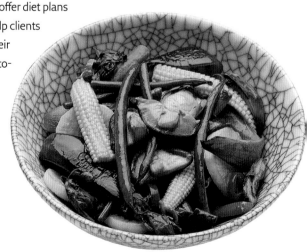

Choose the right diet

Hardly a week goes by without the launch of a new diet, each seeming to offer a completely different approach from previous ones, but even if a plan sounds plausible and appealing, it can be hard to assess its nutritional value and effectiveness.

must know

Unsound claims
Complain to your local trading standards office if you see an advertisement for a slimming plan or a product that seems to make unsound claims.

A healthy diet

The principles of healthy eating, as advocated by most responsible weight loss plans, have not changed much in recent years. So any diet proclaiming it is 'brand new' or 'revolutionary' should be treated with caution; the presentation may be different, or other aspects may be new, but a sound weight loss diet should follow standard, familiar principles. There are other signs that indicate how effective and healthy a diet is likely to be, and to help you decide whether it is the kind of plan you would like to follow. The main features of 'good' and 'bad' diets are listed below.

Good diets

It is important to note the pros and cons to every diet and what may work for one person may not be so suitable for another. Always weigh the pros and cons up together. Good diets will:

Explain that their aim is to create an energy deficit
Successful weight loss plans only work by changing the balance between calories in and calories out. Although they may have different ways of recommending how to achieve the energy deficit, responsible plans make it clear that this is why they work.

Enable you to personalize the plan to suit your lifestyle
The weight loss plan that is most likely to work for you in the long term is one that allows you to enjoy your favourite foods in moderation and that fits in with your everyday life and routine.

Advise you to become more physically active

Many slimming diets focus on food and do not provide specific fitness advice. However, now that exercise is widely accepted as such a key part of losing weight and maintaining weight loss, responsible plans will recommend that slimmers become more active as well as following their eating plan.

Include foods from all the major food groups

Unless you have a specific allergy to a specific food, there are no nutritional benefits, and even some risks, in cutting out any major food group. A healthy diet, even a slimming diet, will include foods from all groups.

Have no 'compulsory' foods and no 'banned' foods

It is certainly possible to lose weight by including compulsory foods in the diet or by banning some foods altogether, without compromising health. In the long term, however, it is only human to rebel against rules and restrictions: refusing to eat compulsory foods or giving in to cravings for banned foods could lead to hunger and bingeing, which are counter-productive to healthy, steady weight loss.

Recommend weight loss of 450-900 g (1-2 lb) a week

As we have seen, this is a steady, achievable rate of weight loss in the long term; initial weight losses on starting a diet may be bigger because of water loss but this should even out eventually.

Offer advice and support through lifestyle change

Many slimmers find maintaining their new, lower weight a real challenge. Responsible weight loss plans recognize this by offering a separate eating plan, or detailed advice, on gradually increasing calorie intake to find a balance that enables the weight to be maintained comfortably over time, emphasizing that the change to healthier eating habits and increased activity must be permanent.

must know

Other resources
Ask at your local health centre about the weight management services that the practice offers or recommends. Check out the qualifications of complementary therapists to ensure they offer the kind of help you feel you need.

Address the issues of motivation and support
Losing weight successfully is more than just following a diet; it requires support and practical advice on adjusting to lifestyle changes that need to become second nature to you so that you are more likely to stick to the plan, and keep the weight off long term. A good weight loss plan will offer support either directly (through meetings, telephone or online advice) or it will provide plenty of information on finding help in order to make the necessary changes in your lifestyle and habits.

Bad diets

Suggest a 'normal' healthy diet is not enough to ensure good health
Some diet plans prey on the fears of the 'worried well' by claiming that it is impossible to eat healthily without taking some supplements or special foods, whether you are trying to lose weight or not. However, this is counter to standard medical advice.

Promise weight loss no matter how much, or what, you eat
Claims that you can lose weight by eating 'as much as you like' are sound as long as the unlimited foods are specified: no one can slim by eating unlimited amounts of absolutely any food.

Claim that you can lose weight from specific areas
When fat is lost, it is lost from all over the body and therefore it is not possible to 'direct' a slimming diet towards a specific place, such as your bottom. It may seem that weight seems to disappear more easily from some areas ('apple' shapes may find their waist shrinks quite quickly, for instance), and exercise can help tone up muscle tissue and boost weight loss, but otherwise it is not possible to spot-reduce.

Promote eating only one type of food or foods with special properties
As we have already seen, different diet plans set about achieving the energy deficit in various ways. Eating only one type of food is a very effective way of reducing overall energy intake, especially if the recommended food is low in calories, such as fruit or eggs. Restricting certain combinations of

foods (such as having a burger with no bread) is another way of making an energy deficit more likely. However, this is the only benefit of following such a limited diet and there may well be health risks that are associated with cutting out specific groups of foods. Also, there are no foods that have the ability to make the body burn fat faster to any significant degree; it is the overall energy intake that counts.

Promise weight loss without dieting or exercise

You may be told that you can lose weight 'without dieting', but read the small print and you are likely to find that the plan in question 'doesn't feel like a diet' because it is filling, or consists of everyday foods. Nonetheless, if you are creating an energy deficit, you are dieting; it is impossible to slim without either reducing your calorie intake or increasing your calorie expenditure – preferably both.

Recommend large doses of vitamin or mineral supplements

A slimming diet which is based on sound healthy eating principles should not normally require any vitamin or mineral supplements to be taken, except in those cases where people may have special dietary needs or restrictions. Nutritionists agree that it is generally much better to get vitamins and minerals from food rather than supplements, so a diet that relies on these may be too restrictive to ensure enough nutrients will be available from the food on offer.

Promise permanent weight loss even when the diet is stopped

Some diets, especially those that claim to boost the metabolism with special foods or supplements, promise that the effect will continue even after the course of treatment or diet plan is finished. However, there is no evidence that this is the case.

Claim to induce substantial weight loss by absorbing fat or calories

There is no scientific evidence that food supplements can prevent the body from absorbing fat or calories in any way that would make a significant contribution to weight loss.

Calorie-counting diets

The balance between calorie intake and expenditure is crucial in gaining, losing or maintaining weight. Slimming plans work by creating a negative balance, or energy deficit, between the calories we take in as food, and the energy we expend in everyday living.

Creating a diet plan

Controlling our energy intake by counting the calories in everything we eat and drink is an extremely logical way to approach the business of losing weight and, moreover, this type of diet is based on sound science.

Calorie counting is also a way of creating a personalized diet plan that is tailored to how much weight you have to lose and how fast you want to lose it. You can do this by calculating your basal metabolic rate (BMR) and working out how many calories you need each day to lose around 1lb to 2lb a week.

Because calorie counting is flexible, you can also ensure that you include your favourite foods in your plan, and it is suitable for people with specific dietary requirements, such as vegetarians. Shopping for a calorie-counting diet is easy as nearly all packaged foods have calorie values on the label and reduced-calorie versions of many branded foods are available.

Problems with calorie counting

Nonetheless, many people find it difficult to stick to calorie-counting diets. One reason is that it is essential to know the calorie value of everything that is eaten or drunk throughout the day, but this can involve a lot of weighing and measuring, which is both time-consuming and difficult to fit in with everyday life. It is also important to plan carefully in order to ensure that the daily calorie allowance includes all the nutrients that are needed for a balanced diet, and that there are enough low-calorie, filling foods to prevent you getting hungry through the day. It would be perfectly possible to lose weight by eating only 1,200 calories' worth of chocolate digestives every day (about 13 biscuits), but this would obviously be nutritionally unwise and very difficult to sustain.

Calorie counting can also become oppressive and can lead to unhelpful feelings about food, such as categorizing certain foods as 'good' or 'bad' depending on their calorie content, feeling guilty about exceeding the daily permissible calorie allowance, or craving high-calorie foods that are limited on the diet plan.

Calorie know-how

Food	Calories per 100 g	Reduced-calorie version per 100 g
Vegetable oil spread	739	390
Plain crisps	546	456
Salad cream	348	194
Natural yogurt	79	41
Cheddar cheese	412	261
Cola	39	0
Pork sausage, grilled	318	229
Tomato soup	55	20
Strawberry jam	261	123

Food	How much is 100 calories?
Vegetable oil	11 g
Milk chocolate	18 g
Bran flakes cereal	31 g
New potato	70 g
Skinless chicken	82 g
White spaghetti, boiled	96 g
Bananas	105 g
Apples	212 g
Lettuce	714 g

Typical day's eating

Breakfast
- 28 g bran flakes (90 cals)
- 100 ml skimmed milk (35 cals)
- Medium banana (110 cals)

Lunch
- 50 g lean roast beef (75 cals)
- Lettuce and tomato slices
- 1 tsp low-fat spread (35 cals)
- 2 slices wholemeal bread from 400 g loaf (160 cals)
- 25 g packet low-fat crisps (120 cals)
- Medium apple (45 cals)

Supper
- 100 g poached salmon fillet (200 cals)
- 200 g jacket potato (160 cals)
- 1 tbsp reduced-calorie mayonnaise (50 cals)
- 225 g steamed broccoli and carrots (80 cals)
- Fruit salad: 1 apple (45 cals), 50 g strawberries (20 cals), 28 g grapes (17 cals)
- 125 g pot virtually fat free toffee yogurt (65 cals)

Drinks
- Water, diet cola, tea and coffee with 500 ml skimmed milk (175 cals)

Snack
- 2 Rich Tea biscuits (90 cals)

Total calories per day: 1,572

Low-carbohydrate diets

At one time over 1,000,000 people in the UK were following the Atkins low-carbohydrate, high-protein diet. These diets are less popular now but the belief that carbohydrates cause weight gain remains, and manufacturers have been quick to launch 'low-carb' products.

What you can eat

The first phase of a low-carb diet turns conventional healthy eating wisdom on its head: it typically includes unlimited lean protein foods such as meat, fish and eggs, plus unlimited fat (including saturated fats such as butter), and virtually no carbohydrates at all – no cereals, no pulses, only three handfuls of vegetables a day and no fruit. This regime can be followed for between 14 days and six months, after which carbohydrates are gradually reintroduced and a maintenance level reached. Vitamin and mineral supplements are recommended to keep the body fully supplied with nutrients during the restrictive phase.

Health risks

Organizations including the Food Standards Agency and the British Dietetic Association (BDA) have expressed concern at the risks of slimming in a way that is counter to all conventional advice on healthy eating. The BDA concluded it could not recommend a high-protein diet as a long-term slimming solution, because of concerns about the possible effects of a high protein intake on the kidneys and on calcium loss, and high levels of saturated fat on the heart. It called for further research on the consequences of a high-protein diet for people who already have weight-related medical conditions.

However, thousands of people who have followed low-carbohydrate diets find they are effective, at least in the short term. Research studies have confirmed that a low-carb diet can produce a quicker short-term weight loss than other slimming diets, but that there is no difference in weight loss after six months.

Promoters of low-carb diets say that they work because there is an overall reduction in digestible energy, i.e. the balance of the diet encourages more calories than usual to be burnt up in digestion, and that deprived of glucose from carbohydrates, the body plunders its fat and protein stores to produce energy from ketones, resulting in quick weight loss.

Sceptics agree that there is an overall reduction in energy because the diet is self-limiting – in other words, there is only so much bacon and eggs, without toast, that can be eaten. And as high-protein diets tend to ban refined carbohydrates, which are generally high in calories, then the energy deficit necessary for weight loss can be achieved.

Protein foods are satiating (filling), which helps to keep hunger at bay, while the production of ketones (essentially a starvation reaction) can also result in a feeling of fullness. Other less pleasant short-term side-effects of ketone production can include bad breath, nausea and dizziness. Constipation can also be a problem on a high-protein diet that is very low in fibre.

Weight gain is possible

Losing weight rapidly without ever feeling hungry sounds too good to be true for slimmers and, in the short term, substantial weight loss, in the form of glycogen and water, is almost inevitable. However, taking the 'unlimited fats' rule to the extreme, it would be possible to overeat on these calorie-dense foods and gain weight.

Typical day's eating

Breakfast
▶ Bacon, sausage and eggs, fried in butter

Lunch
▶ Chicken with salad and sour cream dressing

Dinner
▶ Home-made beefburgers with coleslaw and mayonnaise

Snacks
▶ Chicken wings
▶ 2 Cheddar cheese cubes
▶ Half an avocado

Low-fat diets

Fat is the most calorie-dense food group: each gram has nine calories, compared to four calories for carbohydrate and protein. So if the aim is to create a calorie deficit in your diet, then cutting down on high-fat foods is a good place to start.

Reducing fat intake

Healthy eating guidelines recommend that a maximum of 30 per cent of calories in the diet should come from fat; a low-fat diet for weight loss will typically reduce this to around 20 per cent. However, as usual, the total energy intake is what counts in determining weight loss; it would be possible to gain weight on a low-fat diet just by replacing fatty foods with high-sugar, high-calorie foods, so it is important to keep an eye on the overall balance of the diet, too.

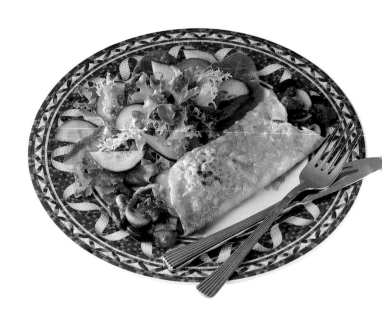

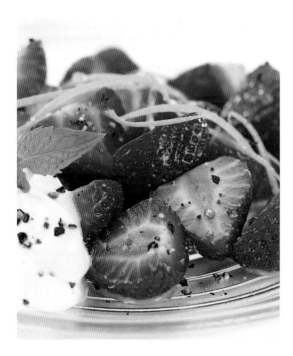

What you can eat

As we have seen, some fats are essential for good health while an excess of others can be harmful. The fats in a low-fat diet should primarily be 'good' monounsaturated or polyunsaturated fats, such as those that are found in olive oil or oily fish, for example. Saturated fats, which are found in foods such as fatty meat and poultry skin or full-fat dairy products, should be kept to a minimum, as should 'trans fats' – hydrogenated vegetable oils, which are most often found in processed foods.

Low-fat diets will control the amount of fat in different ways – for example, by recommending eating only foods that have 4 grams of fat or less per 100 g, or by having a system for counting or measuring fatty foods.

Typical day's eating

Breakfast
▶ Wholemeal toast with scraping of low-fat spread
28 g cereal with skimmed milk
▶ Fresh fruit

Lunch
▶ Jacket potato (no butter) with baked beans
▶ Large salad with fat-free dressing
▶ Very low-fat fruit yogurt

Dinner
▶ Grilled salmon steak
▶ Mediterranean vegetables oven-roasted with 1 dsp olive oil
▶ Couscous made up with water
▶ Large fruit salad with low-fat ice cream

Drinks
▶ Water, diet drinks, tea/coffee with skimmed milk

Snacks
▶ Piece of fruit
▶ Low-fat cereal bar

High-fibre diets

Dietary fibre is essential for good health and many people do not reach the recommended amount of 20–25 g of fibre a day. The promise of a high-fibre diet, providing up to 40 g a day, is that it is very healthy, as well as an effective way of losing weight.

Filling and satisfying

The energy deficit required to lose weight is achieved by filling up on high-fibre foods and measuring portion sizes of other foods, so a weight loss of 450–900 g (1–2 lb) a week should be realistic and achievable. A high-fibre diet fits quite easily into everyday life and is also good for satisfying large appetites, as high-fibre foods are filling, take time to eat, and release glucose slowly into the bloodstream, so that you feel fuller for longer and feel less need for snacks.

What you can eat

All high-fibre diets are based on eating plenty of insoluble fibre – in the form of bran, wholegrain cereals, bread and pasta, brown rice and vegetables – and soluble fibre – fruits, oats and pulses, such as beans, lentils and peas. Because fibre has no calories, high-fibre foods tend to be lower in calories, weight for weight, than other similar foods, so choosing high-fibre foods can automatically reduce your overall energy intake. As fibre is bulky, high-fibre foods are also filling so you're less likely to feel hungry – another way of limiting energy intake.

As well as the high-fibre foods, a high-fibre diet is likely to include lean meat, fish, nuts and seeds. No-sugar muesli, reduced-sugar baked beans on wholemeal toast, and jacket potato with vegetable chilli are typical meals on a high-fibre diet. Fatty and sugary foods are either limited or banned – so you can't pile butter onto your jacket potato or sugar onto your bran flakes, which would send the calorie level soaring. However, treats such as a glass of wine or piece of chocolate are not necessarily ruled out.

Will this work for you?

High-fibre diets aren't suitable for everyone: people with irritable bowel syndrome, for instance, may find that high-bran foods make their symptoms worse. Having trouble adjusting to a sudden increase in fibre intake is much more common; flatulence and stomach-rumbling are notorious side-effects of the early stages of a high-fibre diet, although these should cease to be a problem as the digestive system gears up to cope. Drinking plenty of water is crucial to keep the increased bulk of undigested fibre moving through the bowel and to avoid constipation.

Other possible side-effects of a high-fibre diet could include missing out on nutrients, such as those from fats and protein, if you are eating a great deal of high-fibre cereals and vegetables and not much else. However, in practice this is unlikely as most people choose varieties of lean meat, fish, oil or low-fat spreads to make their high-fibre meals tastier and more interesting.

Bloating

Do be aware that increasing the amount of fibre in the diet without drinking more fluids can result in a feeling of bloating and sluggishness. So make sure that you drink plenty of water.

Typical day's eating

Breakfast
▶ Wholemeal toast with scraping of low-fat spread
▶ Home-made muesli with skimmed milk
▶ Fresh fruit

Lunch
▶ Jacket potato (no butter) with baked beans
▶ Large salad with fat-free dressing
▶ Very low-fat fruit yogurt

Dinner
▶ Lean roast chicken with fat-free gravy
▶ Dry-roast parsnips, new potatoes and peas
▶ Baked apple with dried fruit

Glycaemic index (GI) diets

Diets based on the glycaemic index (GI) have become popular. They focus on the role of carbohydrates (sugary and starchy foods) in the diet, and particularly on the speed at which carbohydrates are digested into glucose and released into the bloodstream.

The concept of the GI

The glycaemic index (GI) is a way of classifying carbohydrates according to how quickly they are digested. Glucose, which is rapidly dispersed into the bloodstream, has a GI rating of 100, while grapefruit has a GI of 14 and spaghetti a GI of 41.

This was developed by nutritionists researching into diabetes, which occurs when the body's ability to produce insulin and regulate glucose is impaired. A key part of managing the condition is to keep glucose levels stable, and researchers found that carbohydrates that are digested slowly cause fewer peaks and troughs in glucose levels than those that release glucose quickly into the blood. People with diabetes are often advised to include low-GI carbohydrates with each meal as part of their treatment plan. People who do not have diabetes do not need help with managing their glucose and insulin levels. But further research into the GI classification has found that it can play an important role in helping to manage weight.

How the GI diet works

The theory behind GI weight loss diets is that filling up on carbohydrates with a low GI helps to control overall energy intake, because they are more likely to keep hunger at bay for longer than other foods. High-GI carbohydrates, by contrast, are believed to produce a short-lived 'sugar rush' followed by a dip in energy and the desire to eat again. Slimmers who are following a low-GI plan are less likely to eat high-sugar, high-fat

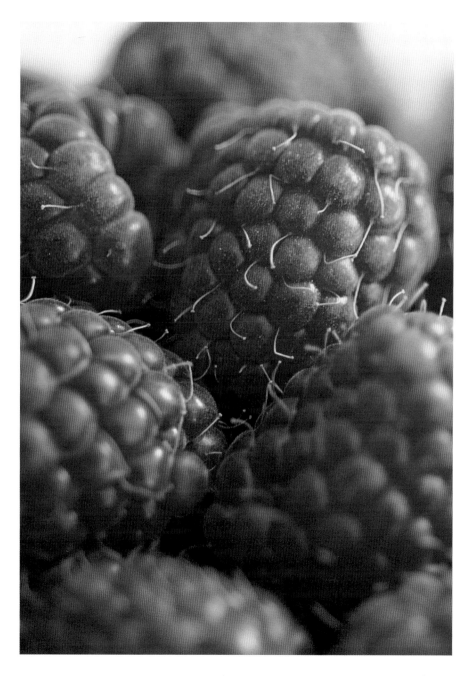

must know

Maintenance
A GI-based plan
can also be used
long-term to
maintain weight,
by sticking to GI
principles but
increasing overall
energy intake.

snacks, and to eat low-fat, high-fibre meals, so that it should be possible to create a calorie deficit resulting in a weight loss at the desirable rate of 450–900 g (1–2 lb) a week.

What you can eat

One reason why the low-GI diet has become very popular with nutritionists is that many of the principles are in line with current thinking on what makes a healthy diet. Low-GI carbohydrates (with a rating below 60) include most fruit and vegetables, wholemeal stoneground bread, porridge, rice and pulses. They are likely to be high in fibre, either soluble or insoluble, which is good for the digestive system and heart health, and many – although not all – are low in sugar and fat.

High GI foods, which are to be limited or avoided on a GI weight loss diet, include white bread, white rice, sugary

Most fresh fruit, like these lemons, has a low GI rating.

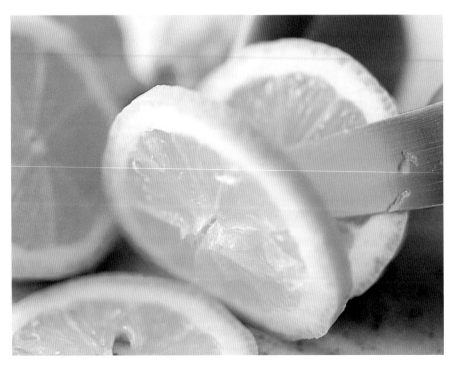

breakfast cereals, and foods made with sugar or white flour such as cakes and biscuits. Processed foods like these are also likely to include saturated fats or trans fats, which need to be limited.

GI and GL

Using GI rating alone as a means of devising a weight-loss plan has practical difficulties. Although many low-GI carbohydrates are low-calorie, others, such as bread, are calorie-dense and are usually eaten sparingly on a weight loss diet.

There are also many factors that influence how quickly the body digests carbohydrate, including the way it is prepared (mashed potato has a higher GI than boiled) and the size of food particles (basmati rice has a lower GI than brown rice). Another factor is the foods eaten at the same time as the carbohydrate.

A development of the GI, the Glycaemic Load (GL) is a way of calculating the overall impact of a food on blood sugar, by multiplying the GI by the amount of carbohydrate in each serving. Foods with a high GL, like potatoes, have a high GI and a high carbohydrate content, and are limited on a GL diet.

Proteins and fats do not have a GI rating because they are not all digested into glucose, as carbohydrates are. However, protein and fats slow down the rate of digestion and lower the overall GI of a meal.

All these complications can make it hard for people to work out exactly what foods to eat and in what combination to create a low-GI, low-calorie, low-fat plan. For these reasons, GI weight loss diets usually have their own way of classifying foods of all kinds so that it is easier to keep an eye on the overall fat and calorie intake.

Typical day's eating

Breakfast
▶ 50 g porridge with water or skimmed milk
▶ 175 g fat-free yogurt
▶ 2 tbsp sliced almonds
▶ 1 orange

Lunch
▶ 1 slice wholemeal bread with fat-free mayonnaise, 120 g lean chicken and salad
▶ Piece of fresh fruit

Dinner
▶ 120 g lean grilled steak
▶ Onions and mushrooms
▶ Broccoli, asparagus and Brussels sprouts
▶ 2–3 boiled new potatoes
▶ Piece of fresh fruit

Snacks
▶ 175 g fat-free fruit yogurt
▶ Piece of fresh fruit
▶ Home-made muesli bar

Drinks
▶ Water; decaffeinated tea or coffee with skimmed milk

Mediterranean diet

The traditional way of eating in the southern Mediterranean has recently been shown to contribute to a longer, healthier life – and following the Greek, Spanish and Italian models can help weight loss, too.

must know

Pros
▶ Eating out is quite easy as Mediterranean-style food is very popular.
▶ Indulgent foods, e.g. olive oil and red wine, are recommended as part of the diet.
▶ A Mediterranean-style diet can help heart health as well as weight loss.

Cons
▶ Portion control is needed to avoid overeating oil-rich food.
▶ A diet designed for sunny climates may not be satisfying to eat in northern Europe.
▶ A traditional Mediterranean lifestyle is very active: doing plenty of exercise is strongly recommended.

What you can eat

The Mediterranean diet is rich in fruit, vegetables and fibre; it contains plenty of starchy foods, usually whole grain varieties; it is high in 'good' monounsaturated and polyunsaturated fats, and low in saturated fat; sugary, processed foods and snacks are eaten very rarely. No wonder it ticks so many boxes as a nutritionist's ideal diet!

Basing a weight-loss diet on Mediterranean principles makes a lot of sense because it is appetizing and filling, as it features many foods that are low in energy density such as lean meat, poultry, fish and seafood; pasta, rice, couscous and potatoes; pulses such as beans and lentils; and fruit and vegetables.

Dairy products are usually eaten as cheese or yogurt rather than milk – and it is easy to shop for low-fat versions of these. Nuts and seeds also feature in the Mediterranean diet, and the main source of fat is olive oil, which is used for cooking as well as dressing foods.

The purest form of Mediterranean diet is found in Crete, but, ironically, obesity is becoming a public health problem in Greece even more rapidly than in the UK. Today, it seems that nowhere in Europe is immune from the influence of the motor car, computer games, convenience food and supermarket snacks.

Health benefits

However, extensive research into the diets of thousands of people who eat along Mediterranean lines shows that they are less likely to have heart attacks or strokes, or to develop certain cancers, than people who eat in the northern European style. No matter how healthy a diet is, it is impossible to escape from the energy equation when trying to lose weight, so calorie control is key to avoid overeating on a Mediterranean-style diet. Even so, choosing to 'eat like a Cretan' can be a helpful basis for a calorie-counting eating plan.

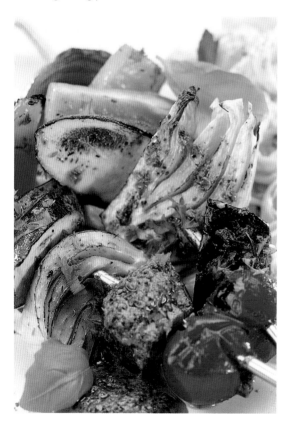

Typical day's eating

Breakfast
▶ Fresh fruit
▶ Bread
▶ Yogurt

Lunch
▶ Salad dressed with olive oil
▶ Bean and tomato soup
▶ Bread

Dinner
▶ Fish stew
▶ Pasta
▶ Roasted vegetables
▶ Piece of cheese
▶ Fresh fruit

Drinks
▶ Water, black coffee
▶ Glass of red wine

Grilled vegetable kebabs: perfect in a Mediterranean-style diet and good for you, too.

Detox diets

Weight loss is only one of the benefits claimed for detox diets: many also promise to improve the skin, reduce cellulite, increase energy levels and promote a feeling of wellbeing.

A body boost

Detox diets are short-term plans, which are designed to be followed for a weekend or even up to a month, after which a maintenance programme may be recommended. The theory behind detox plans is that the body needs an extra boost to eliminate toxins or pollutants that have built up in the tissues; these could range from alcohol, caffeine and cigarette smoke to food additives and residues from medication.

What you can eat

The typical detox diet bans all refined and processed foods, meat and dairy products, caffeine and alcohol, and prescribes meals based on organic wholefoods, fruit and vegetables, nuts, seeds, juices and plenty of water. Many also recommend herbal drinks or vitamin and mineral supplements designed to improve the elimination of waste products through the liver, bowel, kidneys and skin.

Effects of dieting

Detox diets are all very low in calories, which can lead to rapid initial weight loss, mainly of water. This makes them a popular choice as a short-term 'kick-start' for a longer-term slimming plan. Some people who stick to a detox plan also report that they feel more in control and clear-headed. Less welcome side-effects include headaches, nausea, hunger and fatigue. For this reason it is often recommended that people relax at home for the first couple of days of a detox.

The mainstream medical view of detox plans is that they are unnecessary as the body has its own sophisticated and efficient systems for eliminating waste. Cutting down on alcohol and caffeine, giving up smoking, drinking plenty of water, eating fruit and vegetables and exercising regularly should be all the detox help the body needs.

Detox plans

Because they are so low in calories, detox plans are a form of 'crash diet' and should not be followed indefinitely. They are not suitable for pregnant or breastfeeding women or anyone with health problems.

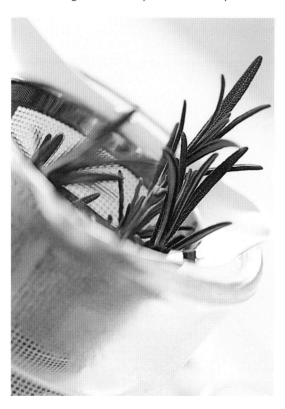

Typical day's eating

Breakfast
▶ Herb tea
▶ Fresh fruit smoothie with oats and honey

Lunch
▶ Clear vegetable soup
▶ Rice cakes
▶ Natural yogurt

Dinner
▶ Grilled tuna
▶ Vegetable stir-fry
▶ Brown rice
▶ Fresh fruit

Drinks
▶ Water
▶ Decaffeinated tea

Snacks
▶ Handful of nuts
▶ Pumpkin seeds

A herbal infusion is one way to start the day on a detox diet.

Diuretic diets

'Diuretic' means 'promoting discharge of urine', and a diuretic diet aims to reduce fluid retention. This can be a serious side-effect of medical conditions such as heart failure and kidney disease, in which case it is treated with prescription drugs.

Diet objectives

People can feel uncomfortably bloated or puffy, or experience weight fluctuations; fluid retention is also one of the main symptoms of pre-menstrual syndrome. A diuretic diet aims to tackle the symptoms of fluid retention that are listed above with weight loss as a welcome side-effect. Some diuretic diets are not promoted as low in calories but will achieve an energy deficit because they limit high-calorie foods.

What you can eat

A diuretic diet may recommend eating lots of foods that are naturally 'watery', such as citrus fruits, melon, and salad vegetables, and diuretic herbs, such as parsley and dandelion. Foods that are limited or banned include carbohydrates, which are digested into glycogen and stored with water in the body, and sodium (salt), as the body will retain water to keep sodium levels at a safe level.

Since a diuretic diet is likely to be very low in calories, water loss and weight loss will result as the body uses glycogen stores for energy. It is still important to drink plenty of water as this will help the digestive system.

As a diuretic diet is usually limited in its variety and low in carbohydrates, it is not designed for long-term weight loss. Some diets recommend diuretic supplements; however, if taken over time these could cause the body to lose nutrients, and should not be necessary.

Food-combining diets

The concept of food combining for health has been around for over 70 years and is based on the premise that proteins and carbohydrate foods must be eaten separately because they 'fight' in the digestive tract and cannot be efficiently digested together.

Science or fiction?

This theory makes no sense from a scientific point of view; if it was correct, it would mean that dairy products and pulses, for example, which contain both protein and carbohydrate, would be inedible. However, the reason food combining has not been consigned to nutrition oblivion is that it has become popular as a weight loss method.

What you can eat

The best known method of food combining is the Hay Diet. It is easy to see how food combining can result in an energy deficit: separating protein and carbohydrate-rich foods means no steak and kidney pie, no bacon sandwiches or fish and chips. Instead, the rules are to eat only fresh fruit or fruit juice before noon, and then to have meals and snacks that consist of either one carbohydrate-rich food with vegetables, or one protein-rich food and vegetables. Fruit must always be eaten alone, and 70 per cent of the food intake must come from 'watery' foods, which tend to be low in calories. Eating processed foods is difficult as they tend to be a mixture of both proteins and carbohydrates, and to fit in with the rules, most meals need to be made from scratch.

Because a food-combining diet is likely to be high in fruit and vegetables and low in refined carbohydrates, sugar and fat, elements of it are in tune with healthy-eating guidelines, but as it is quite restrictive and quirky it could be difficult to sustain.

Crash diets

These will come in many shapes and forms, but the principle is usually the same: to follow a very restricted and unusual plan for a set period of time with the aim of achieving a significant weight loss of, say, up to 3 kg (7 lb) a week or more.

Examples of crash diets

Crash diets are often based on a specific food or range of foods that are claimed (falsely) to speed the weight loss process, such as 'fat-burning' or 'metabolism-boosting' foods. Examples of crash diets would include the boiled egg and grapefruit diet, the banana diet, or the oranges and black coffee diet. Other crash diets use other ways to limit the amount of food that can be eaten, for example by specifying a number of bites per day or a number of spoonfuls per meal.

Short-term effects

As the name suggests, crash diets are so low in calories (typically less than 1,000 calories a day) that short-term rapid weight loss is inevitable. Side-effects though can be extensive, ranging from bad breath to headaches, stomach cramps, dizziness, nausea and tiredness, any or all of which can result from a sudden drastic change to the diet. Hunger is also almost inevitable, which means willpower is required to stick to a crash diet for more than a day or two. Crash diets are also incompatible with a normal social life.

Long-term effects

People who have crash-dieted in the past worry that they may have damaged their metabolism, making it harder to lose weight in future. One reason for this could be that much of the weight lost on a crash diet will be water, and may be regained alarmingly quickly once normal eating is resumed. The evidence suggests that there are unlikely to be long-term physical effects from occasional crash-dieting, although sustained crash-dieting can result in the loss of lean tissue as well as fat, so that when weight is regained the percentage of body fat may increase. The psychological effects of going 'on a diet', failing and then regaining weight, can damage people's self-esteem. Note that crash diets are not suitable for anyone who has a medical condition such as diabetes, high blood pressure, kidney or heart problems. Seek advice from your doctor.

A cup of mint tea could be the highlight of your day on a crash diet, most of which are extremely boring.

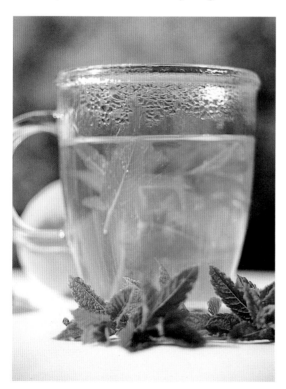

Typical day's eating

A crash diet can really be any diet you follow that dramatically reduces your calorie intake. This 'typical' day of someone on a crash diet may vary in the foods eaten, but will always be sparse and very boring.

Breakfast
► Hot water with lemon
► An orange
► A hard-boiled egg

Lunch
► Tomatoes
► Green salad
► Small piece of cheese

Dinner
► Grilled chicken breast
► Steamed vegetables
► An apple

Drinks
► Water, black coffee

Snacks
► Vegetable sticks

Food intolerance diets

According to research studies, around 25 per cent of people believe they have an allergy or intolerance to certain foods, while only around five per cent have been found to have an allergic response that can be reproduced in a laboratory.

What are they?

Allergy is a medical condition in which the body's immune system responds to an allergen with a range of acute physical symptoms, from itching to vomiting to breathing difficulties. Intolerance is a different condition, which can produce milder symptoms such as bloating, fatigue, or bowel irritation. The most common foods to which people report intolerance are wheat, cow's milk, eggs and sugar.

Weight gain is not usually an effect of allergy or food intolerance; the more extreme symptoms of an allergy are more likely to cause weight loss. Nonetheless, some nutritionists

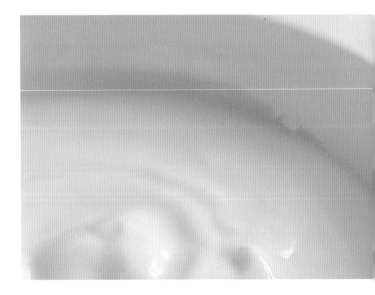

believe that food intolerances can either cause weight gain or make losing weight more difficult.

Diagnosing food intolerances

The methods for diagnosing true allergies are well established, but food intolerance tests are much more open to question; consumer research has found them to be unreliable and contradictory. Sceptics note that the foods that are most often banned on food intolerance diets are cereals, bread, dairy products, sugar and alcohol – all of which tend to be limited on conventional weight-loss diets too. Dietitians have also expressed concern that cutting an entire food group, such as whole grains or dairy products, out of the diet could be damaging to health and should not be undertaken without medical supervision. However, it is best not to ignore troublesome symptoms as occasionally they can indicate some more serious underlying cause; seek qualified medical advice.

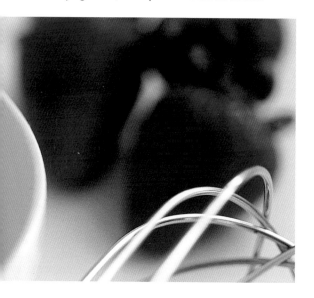

Typical day's eating

What you eat each day on a food intolerance diet depends very much on the foods you are advised to avoid. The aim of a food intolerance diet is not always to lose weight although this may happen if the intolerance symptoms include bloating. This day's eating is typical of someone who is intolerant of the gluten in wheat.

Breakfast
▶ Orange juice
▶ Poached egg on gluten-free toast
▶ Fresh fruit

Lunch
▶ Jacket potato
▶ Cottage cheese
▶ Salad
▶ Fruit yogurt

Dinner
▶ Home-made soup
▶ Grilled chicken
▶ Steamed vegetables
▶ Boiled rice
▶ Fruit salad

Drinks
▶ Tea or coffee with milk
▶ Water

Cow's milk is a common culprit for people with food intolerances. Soya or goat's milk are alternatives.

High-fat diets

Since low-fat diets are the health professionals' recipe for people who wish to lose weight, it might seem very strange indeed that some slimming diets promote exactly the opposite – but they do.

How these diets work

The theory behind all high-fat diets is that by cutting right down on carbohydrates, the body has to use its fat stores for energy, and that this process is speeded up by eating lots of fat – like pouring more oil on a chip-pan fire.

What you can eat

Current healthy-eating guidelines recommend that we should eat a maximum of 30 per cent of our calories from fat per day, with the emphasis on unsaturated fats, such as from olive oil or oily fish. On a high-fat diet, over half of the daily calorie intake may come from fat, and there are no restrictions on saturated fat such as butter or lard.

For slimmers who associate diets with lots of low-fat cottage cheese and no fried foods, a high-fat diet sounds like a dream come true. However, high-fat diets are always low in carbohydrates, and fatty foods without carbohydrates to 'mop them up' are hard to eat in unlimited quantities: a salad that is mainly mayonnaise, or a steak covered in butter, soon becomes unpalatable without bread or potatoes to go with it.

This helps to explain how high-fat diets can achieve the energy deficit that is required for weight loss, and how it is possible to slim while eating seemingly unlimited quantities of fat. As with all weight loss diets, however, the true test is whether they can be sustained in the long term and whether the health of people who follow them improves. There must be question marks over high-fat diets on both these counts.

Anti-cellulite diets

Cellulite is the non-medical name for the lumpy fat that gives skin an 'orange peel' or 'cottage cheese' appearance and slightly swollen texture. It usually affects the thighs and bottom and is mainly a problem for women rather than men. It can worsen with age and can affect slim as well as overweight people.

What causes cellulite?

Various theories exist about what causes cellulite and why it might be different from other types of fat; most common explanations put the blame on a build-up of toxins, a nutritional deficiency or a poorly functioning lymphatic system. For this reason, anti-cellulite diets are often quite similar to detox or diuretic diets, with the emphasis on cleansing the system.

Exercise helps

As cellulite is body fat, most people who are affected find that it improves when they lose weight. Exercise can also be helpful in toning the muscles and defining the shape of the affected areas, so that the texture of the skin looks smoother. However, it may be difficult to eliminate cellulite entirely since it is caused by structural change in the collagen fibres that separate fat cells into clusters, which occurs as the body ages. When weight loss shrinks the fat cells, the dimpled effect will be less visible but the collagen structure remains.

For this reason, it is unlikely that a special anti-cellulite diet will be any more effective than a conventional healthy weight-loss diet in reducing dimpled fat. Cutting down on salt may help as too much salt promotes water retention, which could contribute to the mild swelling seen beneath the skin where cellulite is present.

Pros
▶ An anti-cellulite diet is likely to be low in calories, which will reduce overall energy intake and will produce weight loss.

Cons
▶ There is little evidence that a special diet will be more effective than any other in reducing cellulite.
▶ Extreme diets of any kind are generally harder to stick to and less likely to succeed in the long term.

Body-type diets

These are based on the premise that the physical characteristics with which we are born can help determine the best method for weight loss. One of the best-known diets to take this approach is Ayurveda, which means 'the science of life' in Sanskrit.

Ayurveda

According to traditional Ayurvedic teachings, there are three main body types – Kapha, Pitta and Vata – and six types of taste: astringent, bitter, pungent, salty, sour and sweet. Eating the right combinations of foods and flavours for your body type, and doing the right kind of exercise, can improve your health and wellbeing. A typical day following Ayurvedic principles will consist of no breakfast, a large lunch and a smaller evening meal. The foods that are recommended for weight loss for all body types include grilled chicken and fish, soya protein, whole grains and vegetables.

Blood group diets

These are an alternative option and are based on the idea that different blood groups are more suited to digesting certain nutrients than others. Since the bloodstream is the main carrier of nutrients through the body, eating the wrong kind of foods for an individual blood group can cause weight gain and illness; eating the right kind can result in weight loss and improved general health. A specific diet is prescribed for each blood group, as well as an exercise programme: type O slimmers for instance are advised to have no wheat or grains and to take aerobic exercise; type B slimmers are not allowed to eat chicken or pork and they should play tennis or team sports.

Facial analysis diets

The naturopathic theory that illnesses and stresses can be diagnosed by facial characteristics is taken one step further with facial analysis diets. Practitioners categorise the physical appearance of the face into one of six main types and recommend an eating plan to improve symptoms of underlying health problems and to promote weight loss. Certain foods will be banned and others will be compulsory on a facial analysis diet; for example, people with greasy foreheads, large, open pores and droopy, sagging cheeks should avoid rice, mayonnaise and tomatoes and eat apples, cherries and asparagus.

Body sensitivity diets

People who are confused about whether to cut carbohydrates or count calories are offered help with body sensitivity diets. These are based on the theory that some people are naturally more inclined to gain weight if they eat too many carbohydrates, whereas others are more sensitive to calories from any source. Two eating plans are offered, catering for each sensitivity, both low in calories but one specifically low in carbohydrates.

Body shape diets

Specific help for women is offered by body shape diets, which recommend a different dieting approach for women who have either an 'apple' or a 'pear' shape. This approach goes beyond the well-researched fact that carrying excess fat around the abdomen can increase specific health risks, compared to having surplus fat on the hips and thighs. It suggests that 'apple' and 'pear' shaped women should take up different exercise plans, contraceptive choices and diet strategies depending on their body shape. For example, 'worst foods' for 'pears' include fatty foods, salt and sweets, while 'apples' should avoid foods made with white flour.

Meal replacement diets

These reduce energy intake by replacing one or two meals a day with a low-calorie but nutritionally balanced substitute, such as a milkshake, cereal bar, soup or ready meal. The 'normal' meals eaten follow calorie guidelines and healthy eating principles.

must know

Pros
▶ They are useful for people who eat on the run or who prefer not to decide what to eat at each meal.
▶ Clinical trials suggest meal replacement diets can be effective.

Cons
▶ May be difficult to adjust back to 'normal' eating once target weight is reached.
▶ People who prefer eating real food may find replacement products monotonous.

What are they?

Meal replacement diets can be bought from supermarkets and usually come with information packs including recipes, meal plans, exercise and motivational tips to help people stick to the plan. Some meal replacement products are used in very low-calorie diets (VLCDs), which should only be followed for a short time with medical approval and under supervision.

VLCDs (starting with a calorie allowance of around 500 a day) may be recommended for people who have a severe weight problem, with associated health risks, and who have had difficulty losing weight in more conventional ways. Evidence on VLCDs suggests that while initial rapid weight loss is quicker than with other methods, the long-term results are similar to less drastic methods. However, over-the-counter meal replacement diets are not VLCDs and can be followed without supervision.

The organization Dietitians Working in Obesity Management concluded last year that there is enough evidence to support the use of meal replacements for people who have difficulty controlling portion sizes and/or preparing meals, and who have failed with more

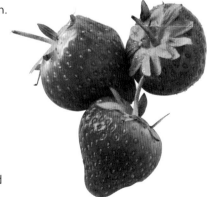

traditional dieting methods. Most of the research, though, has been done with people following clinical controlled trials rather than in everyday life.

Stick to the plan

Commercial meal replacement plans need to be followed exactly to ensure a healthy diet; do not be tempted to create your own version with milkshakes or cereal bars.

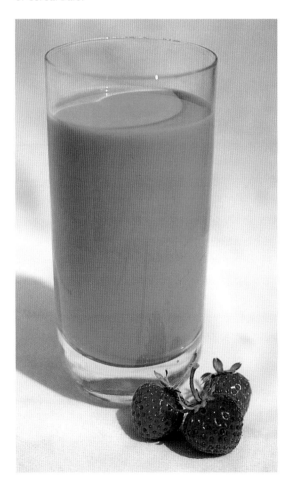

Typical day's eating

Breakfast
▶ Meal replacement product

Lunch
▶ Meal replacement product

Dinner
▶ Balanced meal of up to 600 calories, to include a dessert or small glass of wine, if liked

Snacks
▶ Piece of fruit
▶ Low-fat yogurt
▶ Cereal bar

Other weight loss methods

In addition to the range of different diets that are based on eating plans, as described earlier, there are other aids to losing weight, some of which can be effective for some people.

Hypnotherapy

Described as 'daydreaming with a purpose', hypnotherapy helps to explore the subconscious beliefs and feelings that influence our habits and behaviour. Many of the behaviours that we consider to be 'natural', which will range from basic things like walking to complex concepts such as our preferences for certain foods or activities, are, in fact, learned, although we have forgotten how we learned them.

In adult life, we no longer have to think consciously about these learned beliefs and behaviours, but they are almost impossible to lose or forget. In a hypnotherapy session, the client will become deeply relaxed, in a state similar to that experienced just after waking and just before going to sleep.

In this state, hypnotherapists believe that it is easier for people to connect with their subconscious, which governs ingrained thought patterns and habits. Under hypnosis, people are more able to tune in to their 'inner critic' – the voice that comments on our plans, thoughts and feelings, often in a negative and judgmental way. Having identified the inner critic and how it can affect our self-image and the choices that we make, the client can be encouraged to develop new, more helpful thoughts and habits.

How it works

Hypnotherapy for weight loss will not involve being given diet advice or an exercise programme. Instead, clients are encouraged to think about what might be holding them back from eating healthily or exercise; to challenge those beliefs and to let go of them, in order to create a more positive outlook and confidence in their ability to achieve their goals. A difference may be felt by some people in a single session, or only after several sessions for others. However, not everyone is responsive. Note that hypnotherapy is not usually available on referral from a GP; practitioners see clients on a private basis.

Acupuncture

Based on a form of healing that has been practised in China and the Far East for thousands of years, modern acupuncture focuses on improving the overall wellbeing of the patient. Fine needles, inserted into key points along the body's meridians or energy channels, are intended to stimulate the body's own healing response and to help restore the body's motivating energy, which is known as Qi. The overall aim is to recover the balance between the physical, emotional and spiritual harmony of the individual, which may have been upset by anxiety, stress, poor nutrition, infections or trauma, among other factors.

Stress busting

Acupuncture does not make any specific claims to be a weight loss treatment, and it does not suit everyone, but many people find that it is useful as a way of helping to change their habits, such as giving up smoking. Any treatment that soothes our symptoms of stress or anxiety and improves our feelings of relaxation and wellbeing could be helpful in boosting confidence and the commitment to stick with a healthy eating and exercise campaign.

Acupuncture is not normally available on the NHS and clients do not need to be referred for a private appointment. Before proceeding with any treatment, do check that the practitioner has had at least three years' full time training, or the equivalent.

must know

Pros

▶ If they work as claimed, many over-the-counter treatments could complement the effects of a conventional weight-loss plan.

Cons

▶ These products should never be used as a substitute for, or distraction from, healthy eating and exercise.

▶ They may have unpredictable side-effects and could damage self-confidence if they do not work as claimed.

Over-the-counter treatments

Food supplements, herbal treatments and pills that claim to help weight loss are widely advertised. None is available on prescription in the UK except for orlistat and sibutramine (see opposite), which are the only two drug treatments to have been approved for use by the medical profession here. It is worth bearing this in mind when you are assessing the claims that are made for the various products on offer.

Pills to be avoided for weight loss include diuretics and laxatives, which speed up waste elimination but can have dangerous side-effects when used to excess. Some products claim they can reduce the calorie value of foods eaten by 'binding' or blocking the absorption of fats or starches; others contain substances, such as caffeine, guarana, mateine or ephedrine, which are said to boost metabolism by stimulating the nervous system.

Some herbal products contain iodine-rich substances which stimulate the action of the thyroid gland, whereas fibre pills claim to reduce hunger by making food more filling. Another class of products contains minerals which are said to speed up the metabolism of fat.

Be sceptical

The suppliers of over-the-counter treatments often have research findings to back up their claims, and the active ingredients may have been found to be effective in small trials, or in animal studies, or in specific conditions. However, the dosage and the form of the key ingredients that worked in research may be different in the commercially available version. The most widely advertised treatments come with advice that they should be used together with a calorie-controlled diet and exercise regime; so there really is no fail-safe substitute for long-term lifestyle change if you are to lose weight and keep it off permanently.

Prescription drugs

Two drugs are currently approved in the UK for GPs to prescribe to help with weight loss: orlistat (Xenical) and sibutramine (Reductil). In extensive trials, it has been proved that both these drugs can help people to lose between five and 10 per cent of their body weight and to sustain this loss as long as the treatment is maintained; both drugs have been approved for long-term use.

A third drug, Rimonabant, which works by suppressing the appetite, particularly for fatty and sugary foods, is currently undergoing trials and may become available to the general public within the next year or so.

Orlistat works by blocking the activity of enzymes that digest dietary fat, so that up to 30 per cent of the calories from fat are not absorbed. Sibutramine acts on the central nervous system in the brain, by suppressing feelings of hunger and stimulating the release of energy from food.

Side-effects

Both drugs have side-effects, which may lessen over time. People taking orlistat will need to eat a low-fat diet to avoid diarrhoea, while reported side-effects of sibutramine include constipation, dizziness, dry mouth, insomnia and nausea. Sibutramine also raises blood pressure and pulse rate slightly, so patients need to be monitored regularly.

Doctors are advised to prescribe weight-loss drugs only to people aged between 18 and 65 who are very overweight (BMI 30+ or 28+ if other weight-related risks are high) and who have been following a healthy weight loss and activity programme for the past three to six months without success. Drug treatment should be discontinued if the patient has lost less than five per cent of their body weight after 12 weeks. Sibutramine can be prescribed for up to 12 months at a time, and orlistat for up to 24 months.

must know

Pros
▶ Prescribed medication can help people who need to lose weight for their health and who have found it difficult to do so by conventional methods.

Cons
▶ Medication is an addition to, not a substitute for, any permanent lifestyle change.
▶ The results of drug treatment, while positive, are not significantly better than those to be achieved by committing to a structured healthy eating and exercise plan.

must know

Pros

▶ Research shows
that bariatric
surgery can be very
effective and a life-
saver for people
who urgently need
to lose significant
amounts of weight
for their health.

Cons

▶ Any procedure
under general
anaesthetic will
carry risks.
▶ The dramatic
changes in diet
and lifestyle that
are needed after
surgery are
permanent.
▶ This is an option
to be considered
very carefully and
then only with
specialist support
and advice.

Weight loss surgery

Only a few hundred people in the UK each year have surgery to
help them lose weight, but in the USA over 100,000 operations
are carried out annually. Obesity surgery (known as bariatric
surgery) has been proved to be very effective for people with
life-threatening weight-related conditions, but it is regarded
as a last resort when all other methods of controlling weight,
including prescription drugs, have failed.

Obesity surgery is available privately on referral, and also
on the NHS in the UK, but only for patients who have been
receiving treatment in a specialised hospital obesity clinic.
To be considered for an operation, patients must have a BMI of
40 or more, or 35 or more if they have medical conditions that
would improve with weight loss. They must also be fit enough
to have a general anaesthetic and be psychologically prepared
for the life-changing implications of the operation.

Types of surgical procedure

The following types of surgical procedure are available; they
may be carried out as 'open' or keyhole surgery.

Gastric banding involves the placement of a constricting band
around the top of the stomach to restrict food intake, creating
a small pouch and a narrow passage into the remainder of the
stomach. An inflatable balloon is usually incorporated, which
can be adjusted if necessary after the operation.

Gastroplasty involves partitioning the stomach into two parts,
horizontally or vertically, creating a small segment of the
stomach that fills rapidly with just a few tablespoons of food
and then empties slowly through the digestive system.

Bypass operations involve both restriction of the stomach and
bypassing some of the digestive system, so that fewer calories (and
nutrients) are absorbed from food. There are two options: gastric
bypass and biliopancreatic diversion, which is more extensive.

Obesity surgery patients need specialist dietary advice

before and after the operation and will be monitored for life, to ensure they do not become deficient in nutrients and that there are no complications from the surgery.

Slimming gadgets

Despite the overwhelming evidence that the only way to lose weight is by creating an energy deficit, there is no shortage of products and gadgets that are claimed to bypass this process and produce weight loss with no effort required on the part of the user. Examples include clothes impregnated with substances, which are claimed to burn fat by absorption through the skin; sprays that 'magnify' any calories eaten so that they feel twice as filling; shoe insoles that stimulate energy points in the feet; body creams that dissolve cellulite; rubber bands that are worn on the wrist to control the appetite, and foot patches that slim the body overnight.

Do they work?

These products and others like them are sold over the internet and through advertisements in newspapers and magazines; the evidence the suppliers use to back up their claims is usually less than rigorous, and testimonials from satisfied customers nearly always say that they worked alongside a calorie-cutting diet, so it is not clear whether following the diet alone would have produced the same result.

One exception to this rule may be products that use the sense of smell to help suppress the appetite; trials of a patch scented strongly with vanilla showed that taking a sniff seemed to contribute to the reduction of energy intake as people felt less need to snack. Some slimmers report a similar effect from cleaning their teeth either before a meal or when craving something sweet; it's not clear why this might help but weight loss will depend on the number of calories eaten, not on the effect of individual tastes or smells.

Slimming clubs

The outdated view of slimming clubs is that they offer weekly humiliation in a village hall, with a dragon-like leader nagging her members to lose weight. If this caricature was ever true, it is certainly no longer the case.

What they offer

The slimming clubs of the twenty-first century are sophisticated organizations on a mission to improve Britain's health, and with well over 1,000,000 members between them. In addition to their own eating plans and exercise programmes, slimming clubs offer a wide range of services to their members, ranging from websites and on-line weight loss plans to recipe books, magazines and branded foods. Group leaders, who operate local franchises, are trained in behavioural modification techniques, communication skills and nutrition.

Having worked very hard to lose their 'amateurish' image, slimming clubs are today taking an active part in the public health debate and are finding more favour with the medical

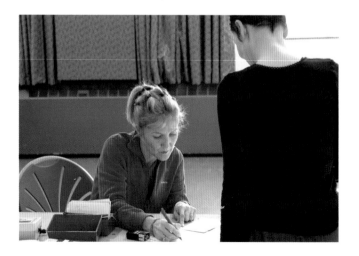

The confidential weekly weigh-in is the focus of many slimming club members' week.

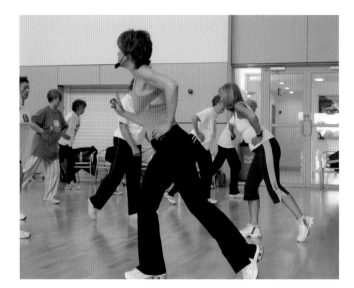

A work-out is on offer for the members of some, but not all, slimming clubs. Choose the style that suits you.

establishment. The main reason for this is that they offer ongoing personal support, which many research studies have found to be a major factor in slimmers' chances of long-term success. Increasingly, the overloaded NHS is turning to commercial slimming organizations to help provide an obesity management service; the three biggest clubs all have schemes offering free or low-cost membership to patients who are referred by their GP.

In the UK, the biggest slimming club networks are Slimming World, Weight Watchers, Rosemary Conley Diet & Fitness Clubs and Scottish Slimmers (in Scotland). All these clubs have eating plans which are designed by nutritionists for good health as well as weight loss. Many smaller, local clubs, however, do not have these resources; if you are in doubt about the eating plan on offer, ask your GP's advice.

One aspect of slimming clubs' old image that is still true is that they are overwhelmingly a female preserve: the ratio of women to men is typically 9:1. However, some clubs do offer men-only groups, and all have a policy of making men welcome.

Rosemary Conley

The Rosemary Conley Diet & Fitness Clubs are run by franchisees who are trained fitness instructors and offer nutritional advice. The Rosemary Conley approach to losing weight is to combine a low-calorie, low-fat diet with 30 minutes' aerobic exercise every day; each weekly meeting includes a workout as well as a weigh-in. A wide range of Rosemary Conley-branded products is available for members to buy, including fitness DVDs, videos, recipe books, pedometers, kitchen equipment and supermarket foods.

The eating plan

Unlike the other big slimming clubs, Rosemary Conley's eating plan does not have its own unique system for classifying foods; members are encouraged to read food labels, count calories and avoid foods that have more than five per cent fat. A typical day's eating consists of breakfast, lunch, dinner, a dessert and one unit of alcohol, if liked. The emphasis is on self-control and carefully monitoring the portion sizes. As an alternative to attending weekly meetings, Rosemary Conley offers a postal membership pack and an online slimming club.

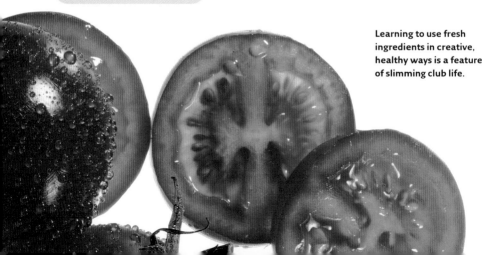

**Learning to use fresh
ingredients in creative,
healthy ways is a feature
of slimming club life.**

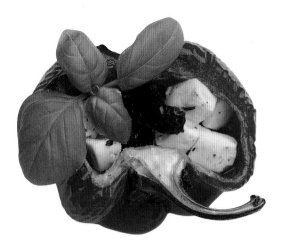

Slimming World

There are three elements to Slimming World's approach to weight loss – an eating plan known as Food Optimising; a scheme called Body Magic that encourages members to be more active; and individual motivation and support within the weekly group setting, a process called Image Therapy.

The eating plan

Food Optimising is based on offering slimmers a wide choice of foods that can be eaten without limit. All these 'Free Foods' are relatively low in calories, weight for weight, and can be eaten to satisfy the appetite while keeping the overall calorie intake low enough to create an energy deficit. No foods are banned and none is compulsory; a balance of nutrients is ensured by 'Healthy Extra' choices in addition to Free Foods, and treats can be counted as part of a daily allowance. Like other slimming clubs, Slimming World prides itself on the warmth and humour of its groups and its non-judgmental, supportive approach to helping members make lifestyle changes. It offers free online support to its members and operates a subscription-based online service – BodyOptimise.

Typical day's eating

On a Slimming World plan you could eat the following:

Breakfast
▶ Poached eggs, grilled mushrooms, tomatoes
▶ 2 small slices wholemeal toast
▶ Fresh fruit

Lunch
▶ Jacket potato, baked beans, 40 g reduced-fat Cheddar cheese, salad, fat-free dressing

Dinner
▶ 85 g grilled tuna steak, pasta, ratatouille
▶ Fresh fruit salad, very low-fat fruit yogurt

Snacks
▶ 25 g packet crisps
▶ 125 ml glass wine
▶ Apple, banana, grapes
▶ 350 ml skimmed milk

Weight Watchers

Weight Watchers' eating plan is called Switch, and it offers two choices. In Full Choice, all foods have a 'Points' value and members can eat whatever they like, as long as they do not exceed their daily maximum Points allowance, which is based on age, starting weight and activity level. No Count allows members three meals a day, which are taken from a long list of foods that need not be weighed or measured, plus a weekly Points allowance for treats and snacks.

On both plans, members are encouraged to devise their own meals along healthy-eating guidelines. Calorie and fat levels are controlled by the Points value allocated to foods; with No Count, foods that can be eaten freely are low in energy

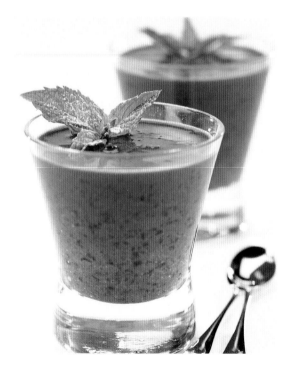

Recipes can help you get clever with low-calorie cooking.

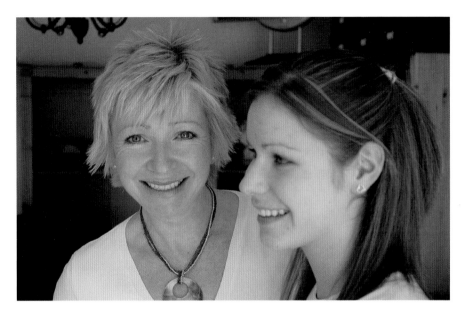

Sharing ups and downs with the group is a key factor in success.

density so are filling while reducing the overall calorie intake. On both choices, members can earn extra Points by becoming more active; this depends on the member's weight and usual activity level.

More than just a slimming club

Weight Watchers is well known as more than just a slimming club because of its range of low-fat and low-calorie branded foods, which are available in supermarkets. At their weekly meetings, members have access to many more products, including a magazine, recipe books, sweets, cereal bars and Points calculators, plus eSource, an online paid-for service to Weight Watchers members.

In the weekly meeting, members will have a confidential weigh-in and will learn about the '10 Winning Habits', based on research conducted among successful Weight Watchers slimmers.

must know

Which club?
A slimming club meeting relies very much on the atmosphere and the group leader's approach. This can vary widely even within the same organization so if you don't get on with one group, try another.

Slimming websites

There are three main types of website about slimming on the internet: sites providing information on weight and health; sites selling slimming products; and interactive sites that offer eating plans and support, like an online version of a slimming club.

Judging a site

Information-only websites are likely to be free to access, but those internet sites that are specifically selling products and interactive services will require a payment or subscription. As the internet operates with a minimum of regulation, there are few guarantees of how useful and effective an individual website might be so you must be sceptical when surfing the web for slimming sites.

And as the internet is a fast-moving world, services can change or even disappear without warning, especially the sites that sell slimming products, such as pills or food supplements. Some of these websites claim to offer drugs that are only available on prescription in the UK, while others make outrageous claims about weight loss without any dieting or exercise. At best, these products could be a waste of money and, at worst, they may be dangerous.

Sponsorship credentials

One way to work out how responsible a web-based service is likely to be is to look at the credentials of the sponsor. Some of the best-designed and well-resourced information sites are backed by the Government, the BBC, health professional associations and charities. These can be very helpful in terms of the tips and information on healthy eating and stepping up activity that they provide, but, inevitably, they lack the element of personal service that the online slimming clubs offer to aspiring dieters.

Motivation and support

The idea of an online slimming club can be appealing for people who do not have the time or the inclination to visit a local group, but would still like a personal service and the opportunity to contact fellow slimmers.

Support is available 24 hours a day, seven days a week, and although there is little research into the success of online slimming services, anecdotal evidence and testimonials suggest that some slimmers find them very motivating and effective. Some of the biggest online slimming clubs are based in the USA, which need not deter British slimmers who accept that some of the branded foods mentioned may not be available in the UK and are happy to work with US weights and measures.

Key checks to make before joining an online slimming club are that personal details such as medical history are asked for and taken into account; that the system is genuinely responsive to information supplied to it – for example, by querying an unusually high weight loss or gain; and that it makes subscribers aware from the outset of any extra costs that may be payable, such as for foods and products, and about the policy on cancellation.

Site quality

One indication of a site's quality is the company it keeps: responsible services will not host advertisements or links for sites selling 'get slim quick' solutions.

Which site?

Major supermarkets and the big slimming clubs are behind some of the best interactive services. As these organizations have their own reputations and standards to maintain, they will offer well-researched information and efficient customer service.

Want to know more?

Take it to the next level...

- ▶ **Creating an energy deficit** 50
- ▶ **Healthy eating and fat** 71
- ▶ **Useful website addresses** 185

Other sources

- ▶ **Books listing the fat, calorie and fibre content of basic and branded foods are useful in working out where your favourites fit in to a specific weight loss plan.**
- ▶ **Healthy-eating cookery books and food websites are full of good ideas for low-fat recipes, cooking and shopping.**
- ▶ **To find a qualified dietitian, see: www.bda.uk.com**
- ▶ **To check out diet claims, see: www.which.com www.quackwatch.org**

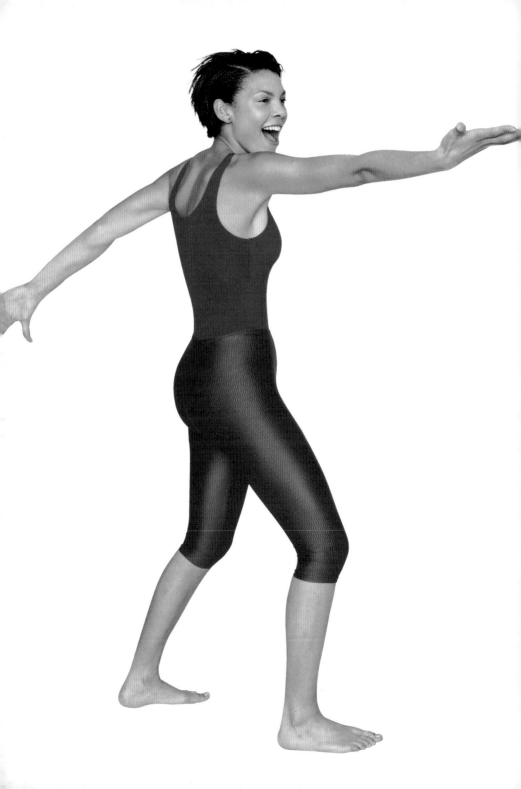

7 Exercise: the energy booster

Activity helps the body burn more calories, but
that is only one of the reasons why combining
a healthy eating plan with following an exercise
programme is the best way to slim and stay
slim. The good news is that getting active need
not mean going to the gym or being sporty;
it is easy to enjoy the benefits of exercise by
making it part of your everyday life.

Move it to lose it

Slimmers who lose weight by changing their diet alone, without becoming more active, are missing out on an opportunity to boost their weight loss, general health and energy levels – as well as having some fun while they are shaping up.

Our sedentary society

In Chapter 3 we saw how the twenty-first century environment can be hostile to people who want to make healthy food choices and control their weight. In the same way, making time to be active can be difficult when many of us have sedentary jobs, drive cars, use labour-saving devices and spend our leisure time watching TV or going out for meals.

Fifty years ago, activity was an essential part of most people's lives; they walked or cycled everywhere, did many household chores by hand, and had physically demanding jobs. Today, it takes effort to build exercise back into our lives.

Surveys have found that between 1975 and 2001, the total miles travelled by foot and bicycle fell by 26 per cent, a difference of 66 miles walked per person per year. Other studies show the number of people choosing active pastimes such as swimming, yoga and keep fit has increased, but not enough to compensate for the overall decrease in activity as part of daily routines.

The result, according to a 2004 report from the Chief Medical Officer (CMO) for England, is that about two-thirds of men and three-quarters of women do less than the level of exercise recommended to maintain health: 30 minutes of moderate activity a day at least five days of the week. One-third of men, and between a third and a half of women, are officially 'sedentary', doing less than 30 minutes of activity per week.

The CMO report concluded that physical inactivity is just as important as smoking and an unhealthy diet in the risk it poses to the nation's health and wellbeing. Making time to be active is important for everyone who wants to live a long and healthy life, but for people who want to lose weight, exercise has a vital role to play. This is because, as we have already seen, the key to losing weight successfully is to create an energy deficit so we expend more calories than we take in as food. Changing your diet to control calorie intake is one side of this energy equation: becoming more active to burn off more calories is the other.

Worth the effort: being active can boost self-esteem.

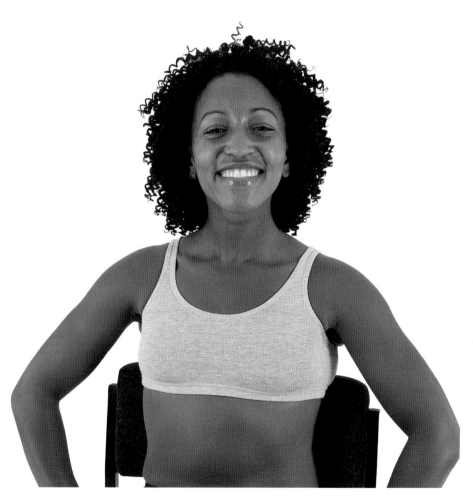

Finding a form of exercise you enjoy is key to being able to make it a habit.

Why exercise?

Every movement we make, from changing the TV channel using the remote control to running a marathon, burns up calories – the table on page 145 shows how many calories are used up in a wide range of activities.

When deciding to lose weight, some people immediately think of exercise as the solution, on the basis that going for a run or a gym workout a few times a week is a more appealing option than changing their diet. However, as we shall see, it takes a great deal of exercise to burn fat by activity alone: to use up around 3,500 calories (the equivalent of a pound of fat), the average person would need to spend nearly seven hours running or dancing energetically.

This is another aspect of the genetic legacy that we have received from our ancestors; survival in an environment where food was scarce ensured that human beings evolved to be very efficient at storing energy and economical in expending it. So while it takes only a few minutes to eat 1,000 calories' worth of food, it takes a lot longer to burn off 1,000 calories in activity.

Losing weight by changing our diet is therefore likely to be a quicker process than by exercising alone, and many people find that they can slim successfully without doing any extra activity at all. All the evidence suggests, however, that people who combine diet and exercise are more successful not just at losing weight, but also at keeping it off, than those who slim by dieting alone.

How exercise helps you slim

One of the best reasons for building activity into a slimming campaign is that it makes it much easier to create the energy deficit required to lose weight. We have seen that, for most people, creating a deficit of 500 calories a day will be enough to

must know

Measuring exercise
There are three ways of measuring the amount of exercise we do:
1 Frequency – how often we do it.
2 Intensity we do it with.
3 Time we devote to it (FIT).
To build activity into a habit, the first step is to increase the frequency of exercise sessions; the second is to increase the time of each session, and the third step should be to build intensity, e.g. by noting how deeply you are breathing and your heart rate.

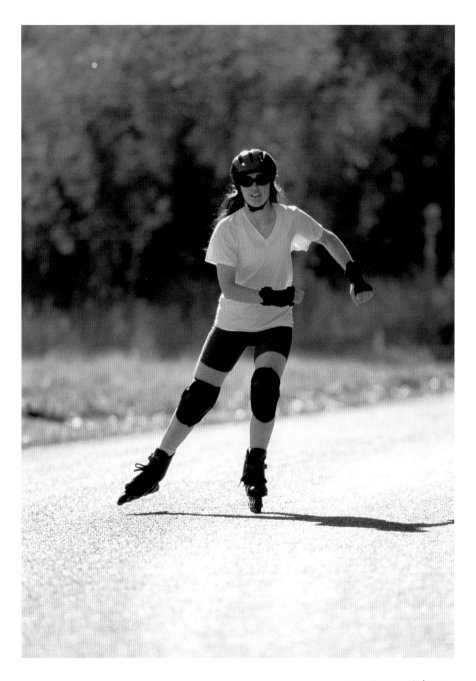

produce a steady weight loss of 450 g (1 lb) per week. This can be achieved either by reducing their food intake by 500 calories or by expending 500 extra calories in exercise – an achievable target, but nevertheless quite challenging.

Altering both sides of the equation – by reducing our calorie intake by 250 a day and increasing our activity by 250 calories' worth a day – has the same effect, but is much more appealing for slimmers who don't want to make drastic changes to their diet or spend hours exercising.

If the only role of exercise were to help create a daily energy deficit, it would be worth doing. However, regular activity has so many benefits, both physical and psychological, that it can truly be said to be the 'secret weapon' in any slimmer's campaign for a slim, healthy body for life.

Boosting metabolism

The most powerful effect of exercise is that it boosts the metabolism and helps the body to become a more efficient burner of energy, both while exercising and at rest. This is because exercise helps to decrease the proportion of fat in the body and increase the proportion of lean muscle tissue. On average, 450 g (1 lb) of body fat needs two calories to maintain itself over 24 hours, while 450 g (1 lb) of muscle burns around 35 calories. So building more lean tissue means that the metabolism ticks over at a higher rate even during sleep.

This helps to explain why people who exercise tend to maintain their weight loss more easily. Slimming by dieting alone reduces body fat but some lean tissue is also lost. Exercising throughout your diet helps you to maintain and build on the proportion of lean tissue, so that the body's metabolic rate can remain stable, even while the total body weight is going down.

must know

Don't worry
People who start an exercise programme having been very inactive could see a small weight gain at first, as the body adjusts to burning off more calories by retaining more water and begins to lose fat and build muscle. It is important not to be put off by this as the increased activity will produce weight loss over time.

The 'feelgood factor'

Strengthening the muscles through regular exercise also helps to tone them and to tighten up any flabby areas, so that the body looks trim and shapely as well as slim.

Another very important effect of exercise is that it can lift our spirits and contribute to a general feeling of wellbeing and confidence. While this does not help weight loss directly, it can be enormously helpful in creating a 'feelgood factor' around losing weight, so that people feel more positive about making healthy food choices, more motivated to continue and more satisfied with their progress.

How exercise boosts health

The 2004 CMO report into exercise and health concluded that adults who are physically active have a 20-30 per cent reduced risk of dying prematurely from any cause, and are half as likely to develop chronic diseases, such as heart disease, stroke, type 2 diabetes and certain cancers, particularly breast cancer, colorectal cancer and lung cancer.

In total, the report identified 20 different conditions that can be prevented or improved by exercise, ranging from depression, osteoporosis, high blood pressure, arthritis and low back pain to sleep disorders, stress and mental impairment in older people.

The report found that exercise can promote good health throughout life, from childhood to old age. It advised that it is never too late to start becoming more active, as the benefits can be felt at any age; conversely, though, it is important to keep up regular activity as the positive effects are lost once inactivity sets in: in other words, 'use it or lose it'.

How much is enough?

The great news for people who don't feel they are 'sporty' or who hated exercise at school is that exercising for good health and weight loss need not mean going to the gym, running or

must know

Get active
The overweight person who walks to the shop instead of driving gets just as much benefit as the runner who shaves a few seconds off his personal best time; every minute spent being active is an achievement, wherever you start from on the road from unfit to fit.

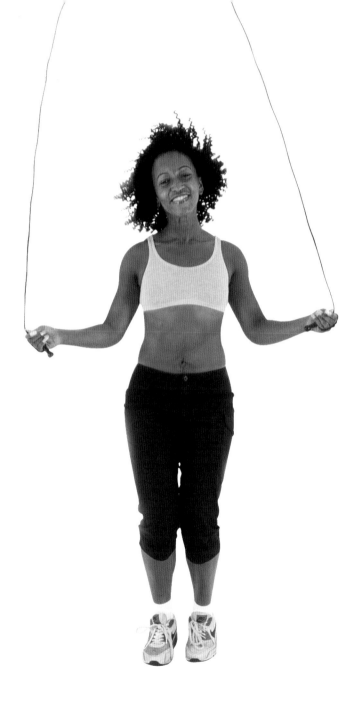

even doing 'proper' exercise at all. The current guidelines for the UK are that for general health, everyone should aim to be moderately active for 30 minutes a day on five days of the week.

For people who want to lose weight, the recommended level of activity is higher, at 45–60 minutes every day. This might sound daunting, but it assumes that the energy deficit is being achieved by exercise alone; as we have already seen, changing the diet as well is an easier way to tip the energy equation without having to do so much – although an hour of exercise a day is a great goal to aim for.

'Moderate activity'

This means exercising at a level at which you are warm and are breathing deeply, with enough breath to hold a conversation but not to sing. The intensity of exercise needed to reach this stage varies widely; for example a very fit person could be chatting away while running or working out in the gym, whereas an unfit person could be breathless just climbing the stairs. The important point to remember is that your body begins to benefit from exercise as soon as you start, and that every minute you spend on being active is an achievement.

What kind of exercise?

The short answer to this question is 'any kind'. Each and every activity that gets the body moving is beneficial to health.

Aerobic exercise

For weight loss, the best kind of exercise is aerobic; it means 'with oxygen' and is the most efficient at burning fat, because it requires a lot of energy. Many research studies have found that aerobic exercise does not have to be in the form of a long, intensive gym workout; people who exercise moderately and regularly for a total of 30 minutes a day lose weight just as successfully as those who spend an hour in the gym less often.

Skipping is intense aerobic activity – a fantastic fat-burner that's fun to practise.

must know

'Passive' exercise machines
These stimulate muscles with electricity or move the limbs mechanically without effort by the user and will not help with weight loss or fat burning. Mobile saunas or clothing that boosts sweating will result only in a short-term loss of fluid and cannot reduce body fat.

Walking is weight-bearing exercise: important for building strong bones.

Resistance exercise and stretching

For all-round fitness and toning, it is worth building two other kinds of activity into your regular routine: resistance exercise and stretching. Aerobic exercise builds stamina but not necessarily muscle strength; resistance exercise means challenging the muscles to grow stronger. This can be done by lifting weights, pushing against resistance bands or balancing on a gymball, which strengthens the core muscles in the stomach and back.

Suppleness and flexibility are also important for fitness, especially as we get older. Stretching classes

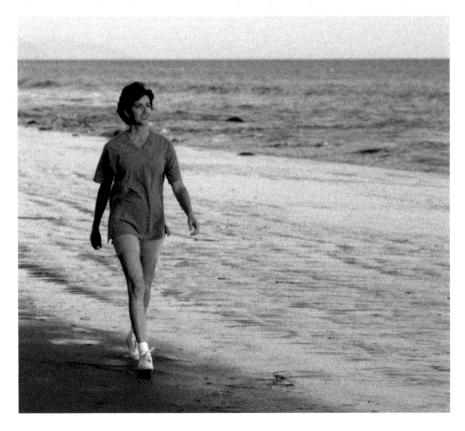

or exercises are usually not aerobic so will not burn fat, but can improve body posture and confidence and reduce the risk of injuries and falls.

Step by step to fitness

Walking is widely recommended as the best all-round exercise for weight loss and it's easy to see why. It's aerobic, so it burns fat; it's weight-bearing, which means it helps maintain bones and build lean tissue, and it's low-impact, which means it carries a low risk of injury. What's more, walking costs nothing, requires no special equipment and can be fitted easily into everyday life: in fact most people do it every day without a second thought.

Any walking is good for health, but for maximum benefits it's best to aim for a 'brisk' pace. 'Brisk' isn't about speed, but about how you feel as you walk: warm but not sweating profusely, breathing more deeply but still able to talk (but not to sing), and aware that your heart is beating faster (but not racing). You might feel this way when walking at 2 mph or at 5 mph, depending on your level of fitness. Generally, a brisk walk for a fit man would be around 4 mph, or 3$^1/_2$ mph for a fit woman.

It takes around 100 calories to walk a mile, so a reasonably fit person could use up about 200 calories on a 30-minute brisk walk – an easy way to help create the energy deficit needed to lose weight, and bringing many health benefits into the bargain.

Which exercise?

Type of Exercise	Benefits	Examples
Aerobic	Burns fat; builds stamina; strengthens heart muscle; increases lung capacity.	Brisk walking; running; dancing; cycling; rowing; skipping; vigorous housework or gardening.
Resistance	Improves strength; boosts metabolism by building muscle; tones and tightens.	Weight machines and free weights; resistance bands; gymball.
Stretching	Improves flexibility, balance and co-ordination; promotes relaxation.	Pilates, tai chi, yoga, stretch classes, body conditioning.

Walk this way

The 'Walking the Way to Health' Initiative recommends a 10-week walking programme (see its website: www.whi.org.uk). The aim is to walk continuously at a brisk pace, but it's important to build up slowly, starting with gentle strolling and pausing if necessary. From week 5 onwards, you can push a bit further by including uphill slopes, increasing your pace, and bending your arms as you swing them to speed you up.

Pedometers

The concept of setting a fitness goal of taking 10,000 steps a day (about five miles) has become a very popular one. Using a pedometer to count every step taken during the day, the aim is to make up the difference between the 'everyday steps' and the 10,000-step goal with brisk walking or other exercise. Many people find this very motivating: there is an extra incentive to leave the car in the furthest corner of the supermarket car park, or to walk up the stairs instead of taking the lift, when you can see your total building up with every step you take.

For weight loss, however, it is important to remember that creating an energy deficit is the key factor: people who are overweight and have active jobs may exceed 10,000 steps a day and yet will still need to change their diet and do more exercise in order to lose weight.

Is the gym for you?

Around 4,000,000 people in the UK belong to a gym, and many gym members find that they are the ideal 'one-stop shop' to provide all the support and services that are needed for getting fit and staying that way.

A typical gym will include facilities for aerobic exercise, such as tennis, squash and swimming, plus gym equipment which provides an aerobic workout, such as treadmills, rowing machines, steppers and cross-trainers. The gym will also feature equipment for resistance training, including weights machines, free weights and gymballs, and there will be studios hosting a wide variety of classes ranging from traditional aerobics to dance sessions, martial arts, circuit training, yoga, body conditioning and relaxation.

Trained staff are on hand to lead classes and to provide individual fitness assessments and advice on using the

Activities tables

These two tables show the amount of calories needed for a wide range of activities, both active and sedentary. The figures are approximate; the actual number of calories expended depends on the weight of the person doing the activity: the heavier the body, the more calories it takes to move around.

Activity	Calories expended in 20 minutes
Dancing – low intensity (walking)	80
Dancing – medium intensity (jogging)	130
Dancing – high intensity (running)	170
Bed-making	100
Cleaning stairs	65
Climbing stairs (72 steps per minute)	95
Climbing stairs (92 steps per minute)	130
Cycling on flat ground ('own speed')	125
Dancing (waltz)	130
Dusting	70
Gardening	110
Golf	100
Knitting	25
Office work (general)	25
Using electric sewing machine	25
Playing cricket	160
Playing pool	65
Playing squash	200
Playing tennis	140
Playing football	140
Playing table tennis	90
Playing cards	40
Running ('own speed')	190
Sitting typing	30
Watching football	40

Source: *Human Energy Requirements: A manual for planners and nutritionists*, by WPT James and EC Scholfield, Oxford University Press (1990). Edited by The Food Commission.

Activity	Calories expended
Using TV remote control	Less than 1
Getting up to change TV channel	3
Sitting, talking on phone, 30 minutes	4
Letting the dog out of the back door	2
Walking the dog, 30 mins	125
Using pre-cut vegetables	0
Washing, cutting vegetables, 15 mins	12
Using automatic car wash	18
Washing and waxing car, 1 hour	300
Using a lift, 3 floors	Less than 1
Walking up three floors	15
Sending email to colleagues, 4 mins	2
Walking and talking to colleague, 4 mins	6
Shopping online, 1 hour	30
Shopping, pushing trolley, 1 hour	200

Source: *Mayo Clinic Proceedings* (77) 2002. Edited by The Food Commission.

must know

The right gym for you
Research shows that the easier a gym is to get to, the more likely it is that people will stay the course, so when choosing a gym, start close to home or work rather than going for the best-known or the most glamorous gym in the area.

equipment; personal training sessions may also be available for an extra fee. Many gyms are also equipped with relaxing extras, such as a beauty spa, saunas, spa pools, a café and family-friendly services like a nursery or children's club.

Nonetheless, thousands of people join gyms each year, full of enthusiasm, only to find that their membership lapses a few months later – or, worse, that they are still paying and never going!

Joining a gym

Before joining a gym, it is important to have a good look round not just to look at the facilities but also to check that they will really meet your needs: for example, are the classes held at convenient times, would you feel comfortable in the changing rooms, do the staff seem friendly and relaxed or is the atmosphere sporty and competitive?

Joining a gym also represents a financial commitment, which many people find motivating; however, spending money each month can be a source of guilt and worry if you find you aren't enjoying the gym or can't go as often as planned. Before signing up, check the policy on cancellation and refunds carefully to see what the financial penalties would be if you wanted to leave; also, work out how often you plan to go, how much each session will cost, and whether this seems like good value to you.

Working out at home

Not everyone enjoys going to the gym or going outside to exercise, and even those who do like the great outdoors find themselves defeated by the weather from time to time. Fortunately, staying at home provides plenty of opportunities to burn calories and tone up, many of which cost little or nothing and are very easy to set up.

Taking part in a regular exercise class can keep your motivation high.

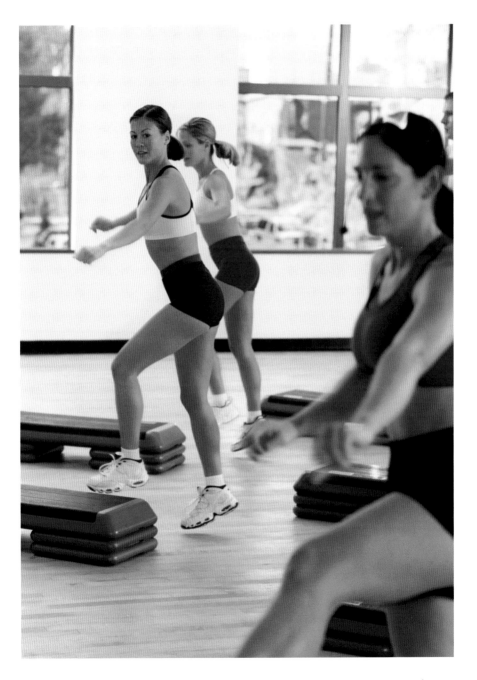

Using your home

You don't necessarily need to buy specialist gym equipment; even everyday equipment around the house can be built into an exercise session:

▶ CD player: dancing to disco anthems, rock 'n' roll classics or chart-toppers for 30 minutes is a great way to get an aerobic workout.

▶ Stairs: walking up and down stairs for 15 minutes is an effective calorie-burner, gets the heart and lungs working and tones the legs.

▶ Cans of beans: these can be used as hand weights to exercise the arms while talking on the phone or waiting for the kettle to boil.

DVDs can help

For a more structured workout, exercise DVDs, books and audio tapes can be great fun and very motivating: it is possible to learn activities like yoga, Pilates and salsa dancing without going to a class, or they can be used to gain confidence before joining a group.

Newcomers to exercise could look for DVDs that have advanced and beginners' versions of the same workout, so that you can take part at your own pace. Building up a collection of DVDs with different styles of workout is a good way to avoid boredom and to focus on different areas of the body, or on aerobic exercise or body conditioning. An exercise mat is often recommended to provide grip for trainers or support for floor work.

must know

Don't be self-conscious
Many people feel they cannot or should not start exercising until they have lost a certain amount of weight – perhaps because they feel uncomfortable or self-conscious or they are just 'too big to exercise'. However, the more you weigh, the more calories it takes to move the body around, so any increase in activity, however small, is always worthwhile.

Specialist equipment

Department stores and sports shops stock all kinds of workout equipment for those who want to take home fitness more seriously. This can range from small items, such as skipping ropes or hand weights, to bigger pieces of equipment like gymballs, rebounders (mini trampolines) and exercise bikes. People who have a bedroom or garage to spare could possibly turn it into a mini-gym; it's possible to buy treadmills, steppers, cross-trainers, rowing machines and weights machines to create a complete home set-up. Before investing in a home gym, do practise on the equipment to check that you would enjoy using it enough to make it worth the money. Take advice on whether your space is suitable, and follow the installation and safety instructions carefully.

Monitor your heart rate

As we have already seen, aerobic exercise strengthens the heart muscle by making it beat faster. To exercise efficiently, the aim should be for the heart to reach its natural 'training zone', so that it is working hard enough to get stronger but not so hard that it causes exhaustion or overheating.

The target heart rate to aim for can be worked out as a percentage of maximum heart rate (MHR). Men can work out their MHR by subtracting their age from 220; women's MHR is 226 minus their age. So the maximum heart rate for a 46-year-old woman would be 180 beats per minute.

According to the British Heart Foundation, the target heart rate for a fast walk or gentle jog should be 65 per cent of MHR,

Yoga can be relaxing or challenging; just choose the level that suits you.

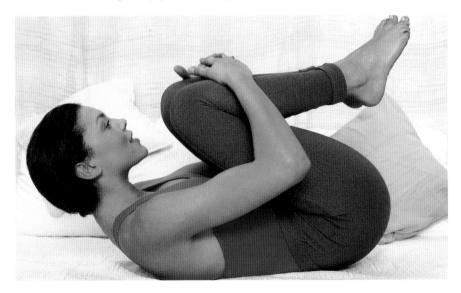

must know

Appetite suppressant
Some slimmers worry that exercising will make them more hungry and liable to overeat, but, generally, vigorous exercise suppresses the appetite in the few hours after activity, and over time, it may help regulate appetite by helping the metabolism work more efficiently.

or 80 per cent of MHR for running. The target heart rate for the 46-year-old woman would therefore be 117 beats per minute when walking quickly or 144 beats per minute when running. The aim of an exercise session should be to build up to the target heart rate and keep working at around this level until it's time to cool down.

Heart rate monitors, worn like a wristwatch, are an easy way of noting your heart rate as you are exercising; some also record the time spent in the target training zone or sound an alarm if the heart rate rises above it.

Top tips for getting fit

▶ To avoid injury, warm up before each exercise session and cool down afterwards. This does not have to mean stretching; the latest advice is that doing a slower version of your chosen activity for a few minutes is just as effective.

▶ Use the weekends to vary your exercise routine and burn

Get the balance right

Beware of using exercise as a way of 'earning' extra calories: studies show that people tend to overestimate the calories they have used up in exercise and underestimate the calories in the food they reward themselves with afterwards! The table below shows how much activity it would take a person weighing 11$\frac{1}{2}$ stone to burn off the calories in a selection of typical post-exercise treats.

Treat	Activity equivalent	Calories
40 g slice carrot cake	30 mins moderate gardening	150
330 ml can cola	30 mins housework	140
Cheeseburger	30 mins playing squash	300
Chocolate digestive biscuit	30 mins bowling	85
Mars bar	30 mins cycling, 10 mph	190
250 ml strawberry smoothie	30 mins window cleaning	120
120 ml glass of wine	30 mins ironing	80

more energy; for example, a hike in hilly countryside or a long walk on a pebbly beach will use more calories than your usual walk round the park.

▶ Think about your key motivation for taking exercise: is it to lose weight, to look better, to improve your health or to find a hobby? Focusing on what you want to achieve can help you find the best form of exercise for you, and stick to it.

▶ Many people find that having an 'exercise buddy' helps them to stay motivated and enjoy their exercise more.

▶ In the first stages of an exercise programme, stop each session while you are still enjoying it and feeling that you could do more. This is much more motivating than overdoing it and feeling exhausted afterwards.

▶ Practise some techniques to remind you to exercise: for example, put your gym kit by the side of the bed, or your walking shoes by the door, or a note on the TV remote control!

▶ Be open-minded about trying new forms of activity; there are so many to choose from and it could be worth trying one or two you don't like in order to find one you love.

▶ Do remember that any form of aerobic activity is beneficial so if time is tight, aim to put more speed and effort into routine jobs such as walking the dog, washing the car or doing the shopping.

▶ Don't give up if you miss an exercise session or two; just get back to your programme as soon as you can.

▶ Book 'exercise time' into your diary and treat it as seriously as you would any other appointment.

▶ Music is a mood-booster, a motivator and a way of making exercise time pass more quickly! Walk or work out to a sound track to make it more fun.

▶ Stay hydrated by drinking water before and after exercise sessions, and take some with you on long walks and on warm days.

want to know more?

Take it to the next level…

▶ **Calculate your basal metabolic rate** 46
▶ **Get motivated** 154
▶ **Useful addresses and websites** 185

Other sources
▶ **Check out your local community centre, library, events website, sports centre or doctor's surgery for details of classes, sports facilities and walking groups.**
▶ **To find a qualified exercise coach, see: www.exerciseregister.org www.nrpt.co.uk**
▶ **Ask your GP if the practice operates an 'exercise on prescription' scheme with local leisure centres.**
▶ **Search for online fitness services to help record progress and offer advice.**
▶ **Invest in a pedometer.**
▶ **Buy a pair of training shoes for running, which offer good support for the feet and ankles, to wear while you are out walking.**
▶ **Visit a DVD library for exercise videos to try at home before you buy.**
▶ **Book in for a fitness assessment at your local gym or leisure centre.**

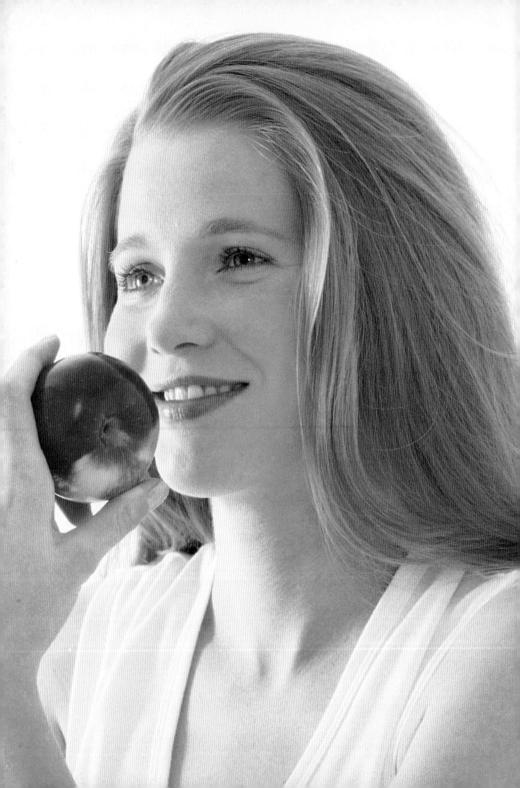

8 Making it happen

Making the lifestyle changes that are needed to lose weight will require motivation – the ability to stay positive and focused for as long as it takes to achieve success. Many slimmers find that keeping their motivation levels high can be the most difficult part of their weight loss journey, but being aware of the obstacles that can arise and planning to overcome them can help to make the path easier.

Confidence and commitment

Research shows that being able to stick with a diet is a bigger factor in success than the diet itself; motivation is the key that can turn a history of failed slimming attempts into a lifetime of success.

Sleep yourself slim
Most people are more likely to snack and comfort-eat when they're tired, but getting a good night's sleep may be more important to weight loss than that: studies show that people who get five hours' sleep or less a night have higher levels of ghrelin (a hunger-inducing hormone) and lower levels of leptin (an appetite-suppressing hormone) than people who sleep for seven or eight hours. As overweight people often have disturbed sleep because of snoring or the more serious condition, sleep apnoea, it is well worth exploring how to overcome insomnia and manage breathing better.

What's my motivation?

Some people are fortunate enough to be able to make a decision to lose weight, find a diet and exercise plan, stick to it like glue and reach their target without any setbacks or disappointments. Unfortunately, they are often the very people who feel they can advise others on how easily they too could achieve success, if only they would follow the same plan with the same willpower.

However, most people's experience of trying to lose weight is very different. They find that willpower alone cannot help them resist the external pressures from our environment to eat unhealthily, or the internal pressures that come from many years of learned behaviour and ingrained responses around food. Even major wake-up calls, such as a diagnosis of weight-related illness or a humiliating experience, are not always enough to prompt the long-lasting lifestyle changes needed to lose weight. Instead, too many slimmers find that despite their best intentions, diets do not last more than a few days. Rather than blame the diet (no matter how faddy or restrictive) they blame themselves and their lack of willpower, and return to their normal eating habits having learned nothing except that they 'can't lose weight' or that 'diets don't work for them'. All too often, this cycle of failure and self-blame continues until it becomes a self-fulfilling prophecy and any attempts at losing weight are abandoned. Yet, as we have already seen, being severely overweight is such a serious health issue that it is vital to find a way out of the cycle.

Why some diets fail

No one should pretend that dieting is a quick or an easy process: that is a recipe for disappointment. One reason dieting attempts fail is that people have unreasonable expectations of how much weight they will lose or the time it will take; another is that they do not allow for the possibility of any setbacks or plan for how they might cope with them.

Nor is it a simple question of setting down a list of motivation rules that will work for everyone. Just as every individual is unique, so every slimming solution needs to be uniquely tailored to suit the individual slimmer's lifestyle, preferences and attitudes – a process that can take time and often proceeds by trial and error. That said, there is enough research and shared experience of how slimmers succeed to be able to put together a general blueprint of effective strategies and techniques that have been shown to help make the journey easier.

Having clear goals and realistic expectations is the first step along the way. Instead of setting off without a route map or an idea of what the destination might look like, it's worth taking some time to explore your hopes for the future, and your fears of what might obstacles might lie in wait on the path to slimming success.

Setting your targets

Setting weight loss targets is a prime example of how people are motivated in different ways. Some slimmers like to have a final target weight set for them and will not rest until they have reached it; others find that having a target to aim for is too daunting, especially if the target seems a long way off or if they have never reached that weight before. And some find that at the slightest sign of being told what to do they rebel like schoolchildren! Nonetheless, having milestones or targets to aim for is worth it, because they help measure progress and also contribute to a sense of achievement: it's a question of picking targets that will be helpful and not counter-productive.

People with a lot of weight to lose often find that setting mini-targets, such as losing 450 g (1 lb) or 900 g (2 lb) a week, or celebrating each 3 kg (7 lb) loss, helps them on a daily and weekly basis, without having to look too far ahead. The final target can then be set when it comes into sight, so that it is motivating and not threatening.

Health professionals often emphasize the target of losing 10 per cent of starting weight, because it is the point at which the health benefits of weight loss start to be noticeable. It is worth celebrating but may not feel so motivating to slimmers who still do not like what they see in the mirror, even if their BMI is no longer in the 'at risk' range. There's a balance between aiming unrealistically for a superslim figure, and settling for an achievable target that doesn't meet the slimmer's true aspirations. The best approach is probably to focus on mini-targets (and other positive targets, such as doing more exercise and making healthy diet changes) and to be flexible in setting the final target weight.

Visualize the benefits

Visualization is a powerful technique which can help people who want to achieve a specific goal. The idea behind it is to picture the situation as it currently is, and then to fast-forward the imagination and build up a vivid picture of how life will look and feel when the goal is achieved.

The first stage

The 'cinema' technique is often used to help visualization. Aim to relax and to set up a blank screen in your mind's eye, on which to project a film of life as it is now, followed by life as it will be when your desired goal is achieved. For weight loss, the first film, of life as it is now, is likely to focus on your behaviour around food, buying clothes, exercising and being in social situations – the more vivid and detailed the scenes, the easier it will be for you to recognize how your life is when your weight is an issue.

Visualizing a free-wheeling lifestyle without a weight problem is the first step to achieving it in reality.

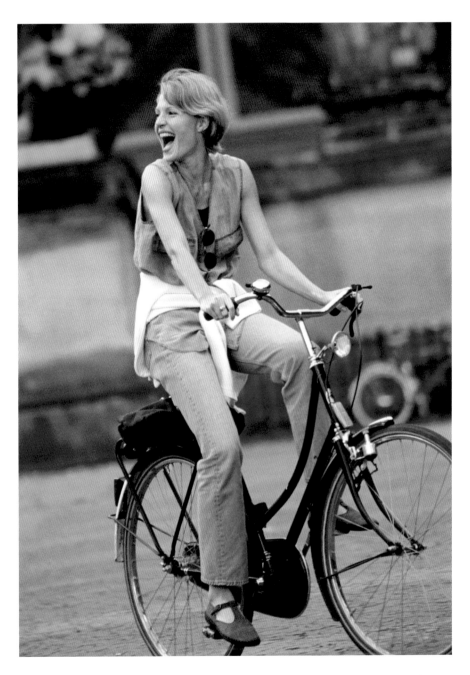

The second stage

This is to turn that film into black and white and to shrink the picture into a corner of the screen. Now it is time to fill the screen with a full-colour film of what life will be like as a slim person. Again, the focus is on our behaviour around food, on exercising, being in social situations and buying clothes. What is happening, how does it feel, what is the slim person doing that is different from the first film?

A successful visualization can help to make positive changes happen before any action has even been taken; picturing life as a slim person can help identify the behaviours and the lifestyle that keep that person slim, and see the steps needed to make the change from imagination to reality.

Explore your fears

No one who starts a weight loss campaign sets out to fail. Yet time after time, slimmers find that they do fail, in spite of their best intentions, and they end up feeling dismayed and puzzled by their behaviour. One reason for this is that they have not established their true motivations for wanting to succeed – or confronted the secret saboteurs that may cause them to fail. These may include fears about the sacrifices that are needed in order for them to lose weight, or worries about the negative consequences of success.

For example, secret fears of being hungry, or of missing out on favourite foods, or of not being able to enjoy a social life, can sabotage a weight loss plan before it's even started as it sets up a negative approach to the whole process. Unexpressed worries that a partner will become jealous or that friends will be resentful of success can stop a slimming campaign in its tracks before the target weight is reached. Sometimes the very thought of starting a diet can be terrifying because the fear of failure is so intense.

must know

Measuring
Taking your measurements can be a motivating way of noting inch loss as well as weight-loss progress. As well as chest, waist and hips, measure the tops of arms, thighs, neck and calves. If you'd rather not know the results in inches or centimetres, use string with knots in it instead of a tape measure. You will be able to see the difference as the inches melt away and you can draw the string tighter.

Conquer your fears

As in many areas of our lives, the best way to conquer fears is to acknowledge and challenge them. Thinking hard about the benefits of changing, and about the consequences of not doing so, can help put worries into perspective, and identify ways to prevent fears becoming reality. For example, choosing a diet that allows plenty of filling foods and treats should ensure that hunger, or the fear of hunger, is not a problem; enlisting the support of our partner and friends can help reassure us that losing weight does not mean that anything else will change.

Spot your danger zones

Every slimmer needs practical strategies to keep them motivated through the inevitable danger zones that can trip up any attempt to stick to healthier eating habits. Keeping a 'food and feelings' diary is a good way to establish personal danger zones and discover whether they are physical or emotional. A common occasion for overeating, for instance, is the first few minutes at home after work, when hunger strikes and it's too early for supper. Another is the garage, where it is all too easy to fill up on some chocolate as well as petrol. Some people find their danger zones have emotional triggers, such as heading for the fridge when they are bored or stressed, or calming themselves with food when they feel elated or upset.

In the long term, everyday pitfalls are more likely to damage a slimming campaign than a special occasion such as a party, yet all too often they are overlooked or not taken seriously as obstacles to be overcome. It may take time for less obvious danger zones to become apparent, especially emotional ones; it is worth establishing whether a pattern exists and, if so, to devise plans to work round it. Taking fresh fruit in the car can help ward off a petrol station snack attack, while having healthy, slimming snacks such as low-fat cheese and crispbreads on hand can fill the gap before supper. Being aware of our personal danger zones is the first step towards gaining control of them.

must know

Plan your meals
Shopping surveys show that we are much more likely to buy healthy foods, such as wholemeal bread and fresh vegetables, at the beginning of the week; high-calorie purchases, such as Chinese takeaways and lager, go up at the weekend. Retailers believe that this is partly because good intentions that shine brightly on Mondays have faded by Friday. Planning the week's meals ahead, to include a majority of healthy foods and a few treats every day, can help to ensure the shopping list stays balanced right through the week.

On the record

Keeping a food diary is an invaluable way of working out how many calories are being eaten each day and of finding out where savings can be made. Studies of successful slimmers show that 'self-monitoring' (the technical term for keeping a diary) is equally useful in helping to lose weight and keep it off. Writing every mouthful down, as it happens and not from memory, is a great way of focusing the mind on the food and drink choices that are being made; and when the week's intake has resulted in a successful weight loss, it's easy to see what went right and how to repeat the success the following week.

A food diary need not be shown to anyone else, and to be effective it should be complete and honest. Some slimmers also find it very helpful to keep private notes or diaries about their feelings and aspirations about losing weight. Creating a 'mood board' or scrapbook of images of how it will feel to be slim, or writing out a list of your problems and then brainstorming on paper how to prioritize them and sorting out the best steps to take, can all help boost your positive feelings and also provide a reminder of the benefits of making changes.

The power of decisions

Decisions are more than just thoughts: they are actions in themselves. Every decision has a consequence, and one important characteristic that successful slimmers have is that they have exercised their 'decision muscle' so that it is strong enough, most of the time at any rate, to make decisions that will help their weight loss campaign rather than hinder it.

Following a healthy eating and exercise plan requires hundreds of daily decisions; some of these are big, obvious choices such as what to have for breakfast; others are much more subtle, such as deciding not to be upset by criticism and reach for the biscuits for comfort, but to channel the hurt and anger into positive action instead. Often, the key to success is

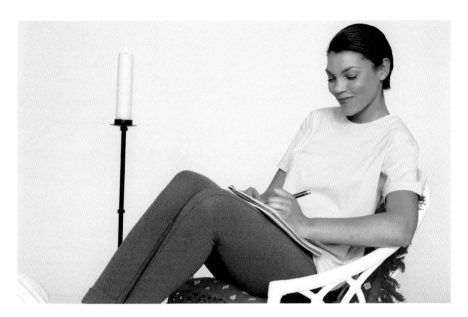

noting the decisions that are almost second nature – such as always driving to work – and to be aware that there are other options, such as taking the bus and walking part of the way.

Taking time to write down your feelings, goals and aspirations about losing weight can be motivating.

Many people will have experienced the rush of positive energy that follows a complete change of scene, such as a holiday. Research has shown that simply asking people to vary their daily routine, by reading a different newspaper or taking another route to work, can result in positive lifestyle changes and weight loss, without a formal diet or exercise plan being needed. The reason seems to be that shaking up daily habits helps the mind to challenge ingrained ways of thinking and sparks the imagination, so that other changes can be more easily accepted and taken on board.

Reviewing the decisions that have led us to our current situation may not be an easy process and it is important not to judge but, instead, to act as a sympathetic observer, prepared to accept the past and build on what has been learned to make more helpful decisions in future.

Get support

Even people who prefer to go it alone in most areas of their life find it hard to make big lifestyle changes, such as losing weight, on their own. Support from their partner, family and friends can be enormously helpful in encouraging progress, sharing in successes and overcoming setbacks. On a practical level, it is also much easier to eat healthily and exercise if other members of the household join in and appreciate the benefits.

Group support

Sometimes, though, only another slimmer can understand the particular pressures of losing weight and that is when belonging to a slimming club or online slimmers' chatroom can help enormously. Studies have found that people lose weight more successfully as part of a group, where behavioural counselling is included as well as advice on diet and exercise, than when following the same plan on their own. Some slimmers find that they need to go outside their circle for the support they need; close family and friends are not always the best people to talk to and may even have their own issues about weight that make it difficult for them to support someone else.

A good slimming club offers a fun evening out as well as vital support.

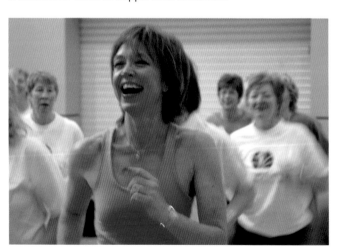

Coping with setbacks

Slimmers who reach their target weight without any setbacks are a tiny minority; most will have days when they over-indulge, weeks when the scales do not budge (or show a gain); or even months when motivation seems to have disappeared for good. In these circumstances, people are usually much tougher on themselves than they would be on anyone else; blaming themselves for being weak, greedy or lazy, and often punishing themselves, either by undoing all the good work they've put in already, or by trying to be super-strict to compensate, and setting themselves up for failure further down the line.

A good support network is one of the best ways to cope with a setback: fellow slimmers understand all too well about disappointment and frustration and can supply practical tips for getting back on track as well as a sympathetic ear and if necessary, a challenge to complacency or self-deception.

Four key points
Whether the setback is a blip or a longer-term problem, four key points (PUFF) can help to stop it becoming a permanent barrier to success.

▶ **Perspective** Recognizing that the weight loss journey is more of a marathon than a sprint can help put setbacks in context. Remembering the successes that have been achieved so far refocuses the mind on the positives of slimming rather than dwelling on the negatives of the setback.

▶ **Understanding** Finding out why the setback has occurred can be key to sorting it out and preventing it happening again. It may be a simple mistake, such as a miscalculation of calories, or a more deep-seated problem, such as fear of success; whatever it is, time spent getting to the root of it will be time well spent.

▶ **Forgiveness** Accepting that no one is perfect and that mistakes can happen to anyone is a big step in the process of drawing a line under a setback and moving on, instead of wasting energy in self-blame and punishment.

▶ **Flexibility** Allowing that there will be times when even the most generous diet plan will not be generous enough, and relaxing enough, to stay positive at these times, can provide valuable reassurance so that even if the occasional battle is lost, victory is still assured in the long term.

Types of support

However, there is more to support than simply having a shoulder to cry on. Different types of support can be helpful at different times:

▶ Information support can be provided by successful slimmers, club leaders or health professionals. They will offer advice and tips on healthy eating or exercise, for instance.

▶ Listening support is invaluable and this can be provided by a good friend who may not be an expert. They will help you to talk through your hopes, fears and problems.

▶ Challenge support can be offered by an exercise buddy or someone who is also losing weight. A spirit of healthy competition can help keep your motivation high.

Diversion tactics

If people saw food just as fuel, it would be much easier to feel in control and behave rationally around it. The truth is that many slimmers have a complex, and not always positive, relationship with food. For some, food is associated with love, rewards and comfort – a link that was forged in babyhood and is hard to break. Others view food as the enemy: a source of guilt and negative emotions, which produces a vicious cycle of cutting back and over-indulging.

People whose relationship with food is so bad that it causes them health problems – such as compulsive bingeing or starving – need professional help to manage the feelings that prompt them to behave in such an extreme way.

Creating natural habits

Most slimmers, however, find that with the right kind of diet, and the right kind of support, they can replace old eating habits and beliefs with others that are more helpful to their health and self-esteem. This is not something that can happen overnight, but it need not take forever either; successful slimmers report that dietary changes can begin to feel like natural habits with a few months of consistent practice.

Positive tactics

There are many positive diversionary tactics that slimmers can employ when a snack attack strikes, so instead of turning to food for comfort, why not try out some of the following ideas?

▶ Exercise: either vigorous activity, which boosts energy levels and suppresses appetite for a couple of hours afterwards, or a relaxing workout like yoga, which helps control the breathing and reduce stress. Sex offers the best of both worlds!

▶ Music: listening, playing, singing or dancing along to music is a recognized stress-buster and occupies the mind.

▶ Pampering: a warm bath, manicure or beauty treatment is a calorie-free luxury.

▶ Laughter: laughing produces the same 'happiness hormones' as exercise and is a welcome escape from everyday worries.

▶ Conversation: picking up the phone for a chat with an upbeat, supportive friend can boost motivation and is a fun way to spend time until a snack attack passes.

▶ 'Safe' food: sometimes diversionary tactics do not work and only food will do. At times like these it is better to have a treat and to enjoy it than to resist a craving and then feel deprived.

▶ Plan ahead: it is easy to plan ahead and to have some low-calorie, comforting foods, such as soups, low-fat desserts, cereal bars, lean cold meat or pasta, on hand to fill up on while ensuring that the weight loss plan stays on track and motivation remains high.

want to know more?

Take it to the next level…

▶ **Find your healthy weight range** 12
▶ **Start a food diary** 48
▶ **Find the right kind of diet for you** 86
▶ **Join a slimming club** 124
▶ **Start a fitness programme** 141
▶ **Useful addresses and websites** 185

Other sources
▶ **Look for self-help books to explore issues such as gaining confidence, setting new goals and conquering fears.**
▶ **Read the slimming magazines for inspiring stories of successful slimmers.**
▶ **Identify all the resources you have for support: ask friends or family to help you, check out websites, or join a gym.**
▶ **Stock up on low-calorie foods, music, DVDs and books as alternative treats and diversions.**
▶ **For help with emotional overeating, see: www.oagb.org.uk**
▶ **For more on setting and reaching goals, see: www.bestyearyet.com**

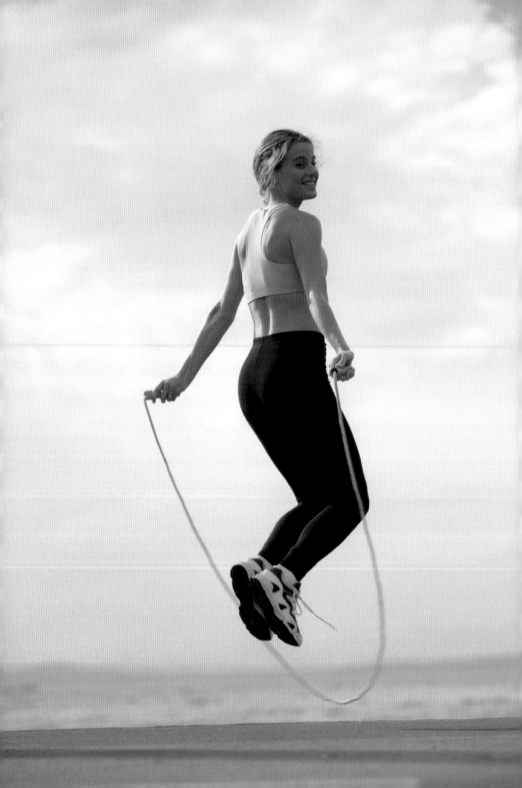

9 Stay slim for life

In order to gain all the benefits of losing weight successfully it is vital to keep up the good work and maintain your new weight, but this can be easier said than done. The secret is to apply the skills that have been learned and to turn them into long-lasting habits, so that staying slim becomes second nature to you.

Make it a habit

Losing weight successfully is a wonderful achievement that deserves to be celebrated – and it is a time to review the lessons that have been learned along the way so that reaching your target weight is not the end of a journey but the beginning of a healthy, slim future.

must know

Change for good
The number of calories needed each day depends partly on body weight; someone who has lost weight will maintain their weight on fewer calories than at the start of their diet. This may not be a big difference, and can be offset by doing more exercise, but it explains why people will gain weight even more quickly than they might expect to if they revert to their pre-slimming eating habits.

It's good to reflect on your success and to think realistically about how you can maintain it.

Take time to take credit

In earlier chapters we have seen that more and more people in the UK are becoming overweight and that a major reason for this is our modern lifestyle, which makes it easy for people to eat too much and hard for them to be active in their everyday life.

Set against this background, overweight people who successfully slim down are exceptional – in their determination to change their habits, take control of their lives and improve their health and wellbeing. Unfortunately, if they keep the weight off, the evidence suggests that they are also very much the exception that proves the rule.

The gloomy figure often quoted is that 95 per cent of slimmers regain weight, which makes it seem that it is hardly worth trying to slim in the first place. It's now thought that the true figure is much more positive: two of the most respected studies into long-term weight loss concluded that between 20 and 30 per cent of slimmers maintain their weight loss over time, rising to 90 per cent of slimmers who adopt certain permanent lifestyle changes (of which more later).

A 20–30 per cent chance of staying slim is much more encouraging than a five per cent chance – but even so, it is clear that long-term success cannot be

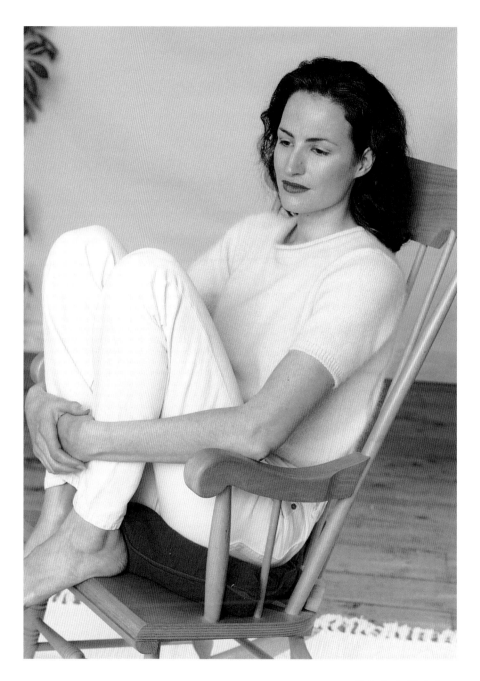

taken for granted. So while reaching your target weight is a genuine cause for celebration, it is also a valuable opportunity to take stock of what has contributed to that success, and to plan for your life as a slim person.

Regaining the balance

Staying slim is all about adjusting from a 'dieting' pattern of eating and exercising to a 'weight maintenance' pattern. The physical adjustment means restoring the balance between calories in and calories out, so that the new weight is maintained. But equally important is the psychological adjustment that is needed to ensure that the healthy habits learned during the dieting phase can still be followed afterwards, even without the regular motivational reward of seeing the pounds melting away.

How long the period of adjustment takes, and how smoothly it runs, will be different for everyone and will to some extent depend on how the weight was lost. Responsible commercial diet plans, especially those offered by slimming clubs and those using meal replacements, provide maintenance

Devising a programme

Following a planned maintenance programme can be a good way of gradually increasing the amount of food eaten each day or each week, until the weight settles at a level that can be easily maintained.

People who have devised their own weight-loss programme will also need to find their own way of adjusting calorie intake that works for them; on a low-fat, calorie-controlled plan for instance the first steps could be to include one or two more servings from the starchy foods or protein group each day, and to monitor weight carefully to make sure that it stays roughly the same from week to week. This is better for health and for satisfying the appetite than to increase calories by eating more fatty, sugary foods or drinking more alcohol.

programmes to enable slimmers to adjust their eating habits over a period of weeks. Slimming clubs may also offer free membership to people who reach their target, as long as they stay within a few pounds of their goal weight.

Culture shock

Slimmers who have lost weight with a very restrictive diet plan may have more difficulties than most in adjusting their eating habits back to normal life. It is human nature for people who have been eating in a faddy way to feel they are 'off the leash' and to relax their eating and exercise habits once they have succeeded. If the weight does not come back on immediately, it can be very tempting to believe that it has gone for good. And by the time the weight gain starts (which it surely will) disillusionment can quickly set in, followed by dismay at the thought of going back to the restrictive regime.

Research shows that although slimmers may have lost weight following very different plans, they tend to adopt similar habits when it comes to maintaining their weight loss – habits

Make sure that your friends and family don't get you back into bad habits.

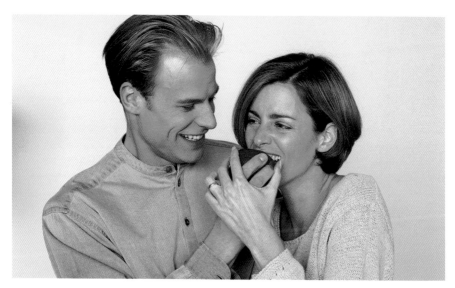

that involve modest rather than drastic changes to
their everyday life. So people who know they have
followed a short-term, drastic plan to lose weight
may need to learn new ways to eat in order to
prepare themselves for a lifetime of healthy eating.

In this case, it is worth comparing the 'dieting
life' with 'normal life' and planning small steps that
can integrate them successfully. For example, it is
a sensible idea to reintroduce 'banned' foods only
gradually rather than bingeing on them; or accept
the occasional invitation to eat out rather than
going out partying every night.

Making a new commitment

One of the key attributes of successful slimmers is
that they have recognized that staying slim involves
a lifetime commitment. Instead of adopting the 'off the diet and fingers
crossed' approach, they incorporate the healthy habits they learned while
losing weight into everyday life, so that they become second nature.

The commitment model

In describing this process, psychologists now talk about the 'commitment
model', and they have found that it has three stages:

1 Psychological commitment

This first stage of committing to a goal involves thinking about it, planning
for it, and challenging any mental obstacles that might get in the way, such
as a belief that it will be difficult, or that we do not deserve to achieve it,
or that the rewards will not be worth the effort.

2 Behavioural commitment

Having become psychologically committed to a goal, the behavioural stage
is to start taking the steps to making it happen – changing habits, finding
strategies to cope with setbacks, taking credit for milestones along the way.

3 Intrinsic commitment

Deciding on a goal and changing behaviour to achieve it can happen quite quickly; the third stage, intrinsic commitment, takes longer because it takes practice and repetition to turn new thought patterns and behaviours into everyday habits. Once intrinsic commitment is achieved, there is no need for external rewards or recognition: the benefits of having achieved the goal are reward enough in themselves.

Note: Many people who slim go through the first two stages of commitment, but give up before reaching the third most valuable stage. Some slimmers manage to lose weight by making the behavioural commitment but never really make the psychological commitment so when they achieve their goal, they lack the self-belief to maintain their success.

Adjusting your habits

Checking through the three stages of the commitment model can be an extremely useful way to start on the adjustment process to a new, slim life. For instance, consider the following:

▶ Under all the excitement of reaching your target weight, there may be fears that the new weight will be impossible to sustain, or that it will be hard to cope with a setback.

▶ Now that family members see that your goal has been achieved, there may be pressure to change your behaviour, such as not going to the gym so often or reverting to your old cooking habits.

▶ The experience of losing weight may not have been as life-changing as you expected; the same old problems and stressful situations still exist. Without the sense of achievement of losing weight each week, there seems little point in committing to change.

Thinking about the possible downsides of losing weight and anticipating the problems that may arise is not being defeatist – it's being a realist. As with any achievement in life, being a successful slimmer has its highs and lows and it is sensible to plan some strategies for managing the lows while enjoying the highs. The commitment to staying slim can be even stronger when it is thought through.

What works, works

Every successful slimmer will have devised their own ways of managing their diet and finding an activity plan that works for them. The one-size-fits-all approach doesn't work when losing weight, so there's no reason why it should work in maintaining weight either. We have already seen that swimming against the 'toxic tide' of our food-rich, activity-poor environment is hard enough; trying to stay slim in a way that doesn't suit our personal preferences or family lifestyle is almost impossible.

People who have found a way that works for them can be evangelistic about it and believe that everyone else should do the same; this creates unnecessary guilt and anxiety among people who feel they aren't 'doing it right'. The fact is that the health benefits of being a normal weight and exercising regularly are such that as long as the overall diet is balanced, the details of daily routine don't matter too much.

What are successful habits?

That said, research into how successful slimmers maintain their weight over a period of time shows that, very broadly, they share a number of habits that seem to have a strong influence on their ability to stay slim.

The two research projects most often referred to are the National Weight Control Registry (NWCR), a database of over 4,000 successful slimmers in the USA, and the Lean Habits Survey, a German study analyzing the behaviour of slimmers and identifying ways of supporting them in making positive behavioural changes.

The members of the NWCR reported that they had lost weight in lots of different ways and for many different reasons, so that there was no clear picture about which weight loss system 'worked best'. However, both NWCR members and Lean Habits Study members said that reducing their portion sizes and/or monitoring their calorie intake, keeping their fat intake

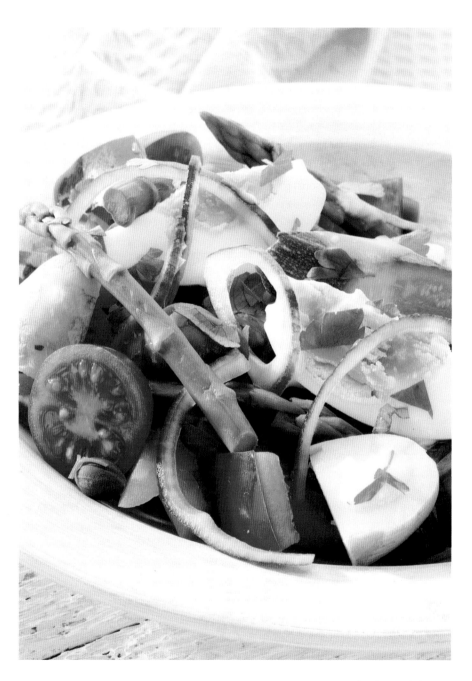

low, and eating plenty of fruit and vegetables and starchy carbohydrates, featured in their weight maintenance plans.

Neither study claims to be the definitive guide to staying slim, but both reveal some other interesting insights that are reassuring news for slimmers who are already on the path to success. These are summarized below.

Eat breakfast

The NWCR found that the vast majority of slimmers who were registered on its database – who to join the Registry must have lost at least 14 kg (30 lb) or more and kept it off for a year – ate breakfast nearly every day.

Nutritionists often stress the importance of breakfast, because it supplies energy to fuel the body for the day ahead. Other research has shown that people who skip breakfast tend to eat more calories in the course of a day, and to snack more on high-fat, high-sugar foods. Many slimmers also report that making time for a healthy breakfast is a sign that they are investing in themselves and in their commitment to change

Good habits start early – so save fry-ups for breakfast for an occasional treat.

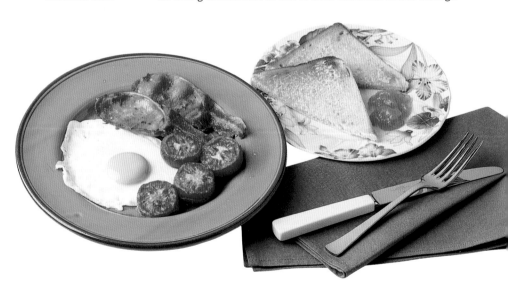

their lifestyle. However, there are no hard and fast rules about this, and maintaining a balance of calories in and calories out over time is the bottom line of staying slim.

Eat regularly

The Lean Habits Study reported that consistent eating patterns, including consuming regular meals and not relying on too many snack foods, was a positive behaviour that helped slimmers to maintain their target weight.

Eating regularly ensures that the blood sugar levels remain stable and do not sink low enough to result in an energy slump, which can make it very tempting to reach for the nearest high-calorie snack between meals. Not being too hungry when it is time to eat also makes it easier to plan the meal and to prepare fresh food, rather than grabbing convenience food that may be quick to cook but isn't very healthy or satisfying.

Exercise regularly

We have already seen that becoming more active plays a vital role in helping weight loss, and both studies found that exercise is equally important in maintaining it.

Members of the NWCR reported that they took on average between 60 and 90 minutes of moderately intensive exercise per day, while the Lean Habits Study found that incorporating exercise into everyday life was a key behaviour that helped people to stay slim.

Slimmers who have exercised while losing weight but do not really enjoy it might be tempted to maintain their target weight by giving up the exercise rather than eating more. This could be counter-productive because exercise

must know

Reaching target weight
Anyone who has lost weight will know that it boosts confidence and self-esteem – and anyone who's regained it knows the sense of failure and guilt that piles on along with the pounds. The rewards of climbing off that diet treadmill can be enormous. Slimmers who feel that they have conquered their weight problem for good report it gives them a huge sense of achievement and self-confidence that spills over into other areas of their lives – very often, reaching their target weight is the spur to realizing further ambitions in their career, hobbies or relationships.

maintains lean muscle tissue, which is a more efficient calorie-burner than fat; without exercise, the proportion of lean tissue in the body could fall over time and make it even harder to maintain weight without cutting calorie intake further. Exercise also boosts our wellbeing and self-esteem, which can reinforce a positive attitude towards eating healthily and staying slim.

Be flexible, with restraint

The Lean Habits Study found that being able to adapt eating behaviour to fit in with different situations, while being aware of controlling overall energy intake, was an important skill in maintaining weight. Other research studies have found that the way that slimmers cope with setbacks can be the difference between success and failure; blips and lapses can occur just as easily in the weight maintenance phase as in the dieting phase, if not more easily. Flexible restraint is also about feeling in enough control around food to make relaxed choices, e.g. on holidays or over Christmas, knowing that control can be taken back again afterwards.

Create a positive eating environment

People who learned to take time to eat meals, sitting down to eat, focusing on the food and savouring each mouthful, found it helpful in managing their weight, the Lean Habits Study found.

Several studies have found that being distracted during a meal, either by watching TV or by chatting to other people, can result in more calories being eaten. Of course, weight loss depends on the total number of calories taken in, rather than the surroundings in which the meals are eaten. But eating while distracted or in a hurry means it is less likely that portion sizes will be monitored; it's easier to forget what food has been eaten, and eating quickly makes it more difficult for the brain to register that the stomach is full.

Manage stress

Being able to cope with different stressful situations was identified by the Lean Habits Study as a skill that was very helpful in being able to maintain weight.

Understanding the emotional triggers that prompt overeating and how to cope with these is a key part of losing weight. Unfortunately, it is impossible to avoid situations that might provoke the impulse to comfort-eat, and sometimes it can be even harder to resist once the target weight has been reached, especially if the emotional triggers that caused the problems in the past, such as a stressful job or an unhappy personal relationship, are still in place.

Losing weight cannot solve all of life's problems and it is unrealistic to expect that it will. However, it can give confidence and a sense of purpose in being able to make changes in other areas of life that need attention.

Monitor weight regularly

The majority of NWCR members reported that they still monitored their weight at least once a week – some did so daily – and that this helped them to stay slim.

Slimmers are not usually encouraged to weigh themselves more than once a week, and this is partly because our weight can fluctuate from day to day and partly because there is more to slimming than just a figure on the scales. However, an important skill in staying slim is being aware of when weight is creeping back on, and having the strategies ready to tackle a weight gain. Knowing how difficult it can be to lose a stone or even half that amount, successful slimmers are ever vigilant in being able to spot a pound or two going on and to prevent them becoming a bigger problem.

want to know more?

Take it to the next level...

▶ **Tips on coping with setbacks** 163
▶ **Metabolic rate** 44
▶ **Low-fat diets** 94
▶ **Healthy eating and the major food groups** 59

Other sources

▶ **Inspire others by sending your success story to the local paper or to a slimming magazine.**
▶ **Set a new target to reinforce your healthy lifestyle: enter a running race, book a yoga holiday or sign up for a massage course.**
▶ **Continue receiving support by giving it: offer to be a slimming buddy to someone who would appreciate regular contact with someone who knows how it feels.**
▶ **Keep cooking and exercise interesting by trying out new foods and recipes, signing up for different dance classes or finding new routes for walks and cycle rides.**
▶ **To join the National Weight Control Registry: www.nwcr.ws**

Personal record planner

Make your own version of this handy food, exercise and feelings diary to plot your progress each week; don't forget to write down all your meals, snacks and drinks at the time you have them.

Day	Breakfast	Lunch	Dinner	Snacks	Drinks	Exercise	Mood
Sunday							
Monday							
Tuesday							
Weds							
Thursday							
Friday							
Saturday							

Plot your progress

Keep your weekly records to remind you of what you do to have a particularly successful week, and to try to work out what you might have done differently if you have a disappointing result.

Weight last week:
Weight today:
Difference:

Total weight loss to date:
Target weight:
Time to target at current rate:

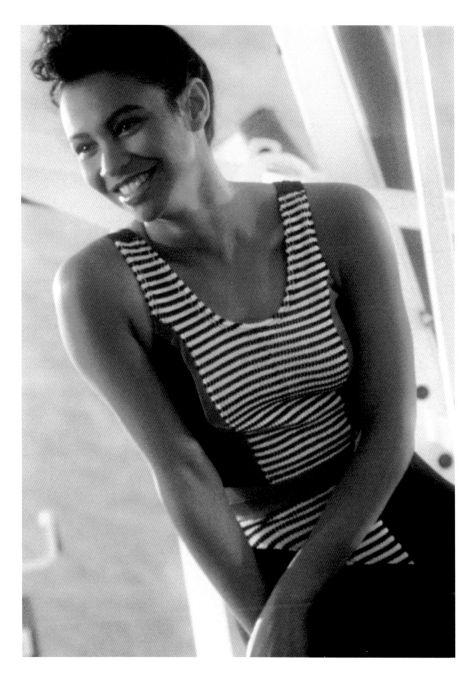

Glossary

Adipose tissue
Another name for fatty tissue.

Amino acids
Substances that form the building blocks of cells and tissues, produced by the digestion of proteins.

Angina pectoris
Chronic pain in the chest caused by shortage of oxygen reaching the heart, because the coronary arteries are narrowed or blocked by a build-up of fatty deposits (atherosclerosis).

Anorexia nervosa
A potentially very serious psychological disorder, mainly affecting young women, who typically go on starvation diets to lose weight in response to a distorted body image and sense of self.

Antioxidants
Beneficial compounds found in fruit and vegetables that help to protect against damage and disease in the body's cells.

Body Mass Index (BMI)
A way of measuring body fat calculated by dividing the weight in kilograms by the height in metres, squared.

Bulimia nervosa
Eating disorder that is physically and psychologically damaging, which typically involves bingeing then vomiting or purging in a bid to lose weight or to maintain a slim figure.

Calorie
Amount of heat required to raise the temperature of 1 gram of water by 1°C; the unit most commonly used to measure the amount of energy in foods.

Carbohydrates
Major food group that consists of two main types: sugars and starches.

Cholesterol
Substance found in blood and all the body's cells; low density lipoprotein (LDL) cholesterol is known as 'bad' cholesterol because high levels indicate a risk of heart disease; high density lipoprotein (HDL) cholesterol is 'good' because it protects against heart disease.

Colonic irrigation
Treatment using quantities of water to flush out and 'cleanse' the colon (large intestine), often recommended during detox plans.

Mainstream medical opinion is that this is only necessary in specific cases, e.g. severe constipation.

Co-morbidity
A medical condition that exists alongside another one, increasing the overall risk to health, eg diabetes and obesity.

Diabesity
Term coined to describe the modern phenomenon of the growing link between obesity and people developing diabetes.

Diabetes mellitus
Medical condition in which the body either fails to produce insulin that's needed to regulate blood sugar levels, or the function of the insulin that is produced is impaired. Type 1 diabetes is often inherited and may be triggered by an external factor such as a virus; type 2 diabetes is often called 'late onset' because it traditionally develops in over-40s and is linked to lifestyle, including weight.

Energy density
Term used to describe the amount of calories in a food relative to its weight; vegetables for example are low in energy density while chocolate is highly energy-dense.

Enzyme
Body chemical that dissolves food at different stages of the digestive process.

Essential fatty acids
Fats that the body cannot make for itself but must take in from food. Fatty acids such as omega-3 are helpful for heart health and in building bones.

Fibre
Substance found in carbohydrate-rich foods that is not digested and so helps food pass through the gut. Soluble fibre (in oats and fruit) helps to regulate the cholesterol level in the blood.

Gall-bladder
Organ that stores bile, which is made in the liver and is used to help the digestion of fats.

Glucose
Product of the digestion of carbohydrates, used by the body as the most readily available source of energy.

Glycogen
The main storage form of glucose in the muscles and the liver.

Glycaemic Index (GI)
Method of classifying carbohydrate-rich foods according to how quickly they release glucose into the bloodstream.

Glycaemic Load (GL)
Refinement of the Glycaemic Index that also takes into account how much carbohydrate a particular food contains per serving.

Glycerol
Substance produced when fats are digested.

Hormone
Substance produced by an endocrine gland (such as the thyroid, testes or pancreas) that regulates the way in which an individual organ operates. A hormone imbalance in a particular organ can cause a metabolic disorder.

Hypertension
Excessively high blood pressure.

Insulin
Hormone produced in the pancreas that regulates glucose levels in the blood.

Ketosis
State that occurs when the body is starved of readily-available glucose from carbohydrates and digests fat from the body cells. A side-effect is the production of ketones, which smell like acetone on the breath.

Liposuction
Medical procedure to remove fat from under the skin by suction; mainly performed for cosmetic reasons.

Macronutrient
Term used to describe the major food groups such as proteins and carbohydrates.

Mesotherapy
Cosmetic treatment to dissolve fat under the skin by injecting soy lecithin.

Metabolism
All the chemical changes that take place within a cell or an organ in order for it to function.

Micronutrient
Term used to describe food components that are needed in very small quantities, such as vitamins and minerals.

'Negative calories'
Term coined to describe a diet fad in which certain foods were claimed to be so low in calories that digesting them expended more energy than they contained. There is no scientific basis for this.

Obese
Medical term for people whose Body Mass Index is over 30; indicates increased risk to health. The word comes from the Latin, meaning 'on account of having eaten'.

Glossary

Obesogen
Term coined by researchers to describe the factors in the modern environment that encourage overeating or a sedentary lifestyle, e.g. escalators, fast food restaurants, motorways, 24-hour supermarkets.

Oedema
Swelling or puffiness caused by retention or build-up of fluids in the body.

Osteoporosis
Medical condition in which bone mass is lost, caused by lack of calcium, lack of weight-bearing exercise, and ageing, which leads to bones breaking easily and to disability. Women are affected more than men.

Phytochemicals
Substances found in tiny quantities in plants that may be beneficial to health. Examples are lycopene (which gives tomatoes their colour) and flavonoids (found in tea and apples).

Polycystic Ovarian Syndrome (PCOS)
Collection of hormone-related symptoms in women, including hairiness and fertility problems, which is linked to insulin resistance and difficulties in managing weight.

Prader-Willi Syndrome
Rare genetic condition that affects the appetite, causing sufferers to eat uncontrollably and leading to severe obesity.

Protein
Major food group found in many types of foods; protein is digested into amino acids, which are used to repair and build body tissues.

Saturated fats
Fats, mainly of animal origin, that are solid at room temperature. A diet high in saturated fats is associated with increased risk of heart disease.

Sleep apnoea
Distressing and potentially serious condition in which the airway is repeatedly blocked during sleep by pressure from the neck: is often treated with equipment such as a mask to help with breathing, but symptoms can be improved by losing weight.

Sodium
The mineral in salt (sodium chloride) that affects blood pressure and regulates fluid in the body.

Thyroid gland
Endocrine gland in the neck that produces the hormone thyroxine, which regulates the level of activity in the body's cells. Hypothyroidism (an underactive thyroid) can reduce the body's metabolic rate.

Trans fatty acids
Fats that have been processed (hydrogenated) to turn a vegetable oil into a solid fat for ease of use. Like saturated fats, too many trans fats in the diet are associated with increased risk to heart health.

Triglycerides
The form in which digested fats are present in the body; triglyceride levels in the blood are one of the factors measured to assess weight-related health risk.

Unsaturated fats
Fats, mainly of plant origin, that are liquid at room temperature. Both mono- and polyunsaturated fats are thought to be more helpful to heart health than saturated fats.

Need to know more?

Charities and support groups

Amarant Trust
80 Lambeth Road
London
SE1 7PW
tel: 01293 413000
www.amarantmenopausetrust.org.uk

Blood Pressure Association
60 Cranmer Terrace
London
SW17 0QS
tel: 020 8772 4994
www.bpassoc.org.uk

British Heart Foundation
14 Fitzhardinge Street
London
W1H 6DH
Heart info line: 0845 070 80 70
www.bhf.org.uk

Cancer Research UK
PO Box 123
Lincoln's Inn Fields
London
WC2A 3PX
tel: 020 7242 0200
www.cancer.org.uk

Diabetes UK
10 Parkway
London
NW1 7AA
tel: 020 7424 1000
www.diabetes.org.uk

Eating Disorders Association
103 Prince of Wales Road
Norwich
NR1 1DW
tel: 0845 634 1414
www.edauk.com

Overeaters Anonymous
PO Box 19
Stretford
Manchester
M32 9EB
tel: 07000 784985
www.oagb.org.uk

TOAST (The Obesity Awareness & Solutions Trust)
The Latton Bush Centre
Southern Way
Harlow,
Essex
CM18 7BL
Helpline: 0845 0450225
www.toast-uk.org

Verity (PCOS)
Unit AS 20.01
The Aberdeen Centre
22–24 Highbury Grove
London
N5 2EA
www.verity-pcos.org.uk

Weight Concern
Brook House
2–6 Torrington Place
London
WC1E 7HN
www.weightconcern.com

Diet methods

The Cambridge Diet
tel: 01536 403344
www.cambridge-diet.com

Rick Gallop's GI Diet
www.gidiet.com

Glycemic Index News
www.glycemicindex.com

Herbalife
tel: 01895 819000
www.herbalife.com

LighterLife
08700 664 747
www.lighterlife.com

Slim-Fast
tel: 0845 600 1311
www.slimfast.co.uk

Food Organizations

The Food Commission
94 White Lion Street
London N1 9PF
tel: 020 7837 2250
www.foodcomm.org.uk

Foodfitness
Food & Drink Federation
6 Catherine Street
London WC2B 5JJ
tel: 020 7836 2460
www.foodfitness.org.uk

Vegetarian Society
Parkdale, Dunham Road
Altrincham, Cheshire WA14 4QG
tel: 0161 925 2000
www.vegsoc.org

Government and NHS organizations

Food Standards Agency
Aviation House
125 Kingsway
London WC2B 6NH
tel: 020 7276 8000
www.food.gov.uk

NHS Direct
0845 46 47
www.nhsdirect.nhs.uk

**National Institute of Health
and Clinical Excellence**
www.nice.org.uk

Prodigy
(National Health Service treatment
guidance)
www.prodigy.nhs.uk

Independent health websites

www.besttreatments.co.uk
www.howsyourdrink.org.uk
www.malehealth.co.uk
www.netdoctor.co.uk

Professional bodies

British Acupuncture Council
63 Jeddo Road
London W12 9HQ
tel: 020 8735 0400
www.acupuncture.org.uk

**British Association for Nutritional
Therapy**
27 Old Gloucester Street
London WC1N 3XX
tel: 08706 061284
www.bant.org.uk

British Dietetic Association
5th Floor Charles House
Great Charles Street
Queensway, Birmingham B3 3HT
tel: 0121 200 8080
www.bda.uk.com
www.bdaweightwise.com

British Nutrition Foundation
High Holborn House
52–54 High Holborn
London WC1V 6RQ
tel: 020 7404 6504
www.nutrition.org.uk

General Hypnotherapy Register
PO Box 204
Lymington SO41 6WP
tel: 01590 683770
www.general-hypnotherapy-
register.com

**National Obesity Forum/Waistwatch
Action**
PO Box 6625
Nottingham NG2 5PA
www.nationalobesityforum.org

Self-help resources
www.bestyearyet.com
www.beyondchocolate.co.uk
www.EasyPeasyWay.com
www.eatingless.com
www.georgiafoster.com

Slimming clubs

Rosemary Conley Diet & Fitness Clubs
Quorn House
Meeting Street
Quorn
Leics LE12 8EX
Tel: 01509 620222
www.rosemary-conley.co.uk

Scottish Slimmers
Weight Management (UK) Ltd
47 St Mary's Court
Huntly Street
Aberdeen AB10 1TH
Tel: 0800 362636
www.positive-eating.com

Slimming World
Clover Nook Road
Somercotes
Alfreton
Derbyshire
DE55 4RF
Tel: 08700 75 46 66
www.slimming-world.com

Weight Watchers UK Ltd
Millennium House
Ludlow Road
Maidenhead
Berkshire SL6 2SL
0845 345 1500
www.weightwatchers.co.uk

Slimming websites

www.bodyoptimise.com
www.cafeslim.co.uk
www.slimwithRosemary.com
www.tescodiets.co.uk
www.vitaline-slimming.com
www.weightlossresources.com
www.yourdietline.com

Sport and fitness organizations

The Countryside Agency
Walking The Way To Health Initiative
01242 533258
www.whi.org.uk

National Register of Personal Trainers
Tel: 0870 200 6010
www.nrpt.co.uk

The Ramblers' Association
2nd Floor, 89 Albert Embankment,
London SE1 7TW
Tel 020 7339 8500
www.ramblers.org.uk

Register of Exercise Professionals
Tel: 020 8686 6464
www.exerciseregister.org

Sport England
www.sportengland.com

Further reading

Books

Best Medicine Weight Management, editor Dr George Kassianos (CSF Medical Communications Ltd)
Body Foods for Life, Jane Clarke (Orion)
Carol Vorderman's Detox for Life: The 28 Day Detox Diet and Beyond, Carol Vorderman (Virgin Books)
The Calorie, Carb and Fat Bible, Dr Jeremy Sims and Tracey Walton (Weight Loss Resources)
The Composition of Foods, McCance and Widdowson (Royal Society of Chemistry)
Eating Less, Gillian Riley, Vermilion.
Manual of Nutrition (MAFF, The Stationery Office)
Gem Calorie Counter (HarperCollins)
Gem Carb Counter (HarperCollins)
Gem GI Guide (HarperCollins)
Gem GL Guide (HarperCollins)
GI Diet, Rick Gallop (Virgin Books)
The Mediterranean Diet (revised and updated), Marissa Cloutier and Eve Adamson (Avon Books)
need to know? Low GI/GL Diet (HarperCollins)
Picture Perfect Weight Loss, Dr Howard M. Shapiro (Rodale International)
The Real Woman's Personal Trainer, Sam Murphy (Kyle Cathie)
The Step Counter Diet, Joanna Hall (Thorsons)
System S, Sally Ann Voak and Professor Anne De Looy (Michael O'Mara Books Ltd)
What Makes My Blood Glucose Levels Go Up and Down?, Dr Jennie Brand-Miller, Kaye Foster-Powell, David Mendosa (Vermilion)

Magazines

Boost! (Scottish Slimmers, Weight Management (UK) Ltd)
Health & Fitness (Nexus Publishing)
Men's Health (National Magazine Company/Rodale)
Rosemary Conley Diet & Fitness (Quorn House Publishing Ltd)
Runner's World (National Magazine Company/Rodale)
Slimmer, healthier, fitter! (Aceville Publications)
Slimming (Emap Esprit)
Slimming World Magazine (Miles-Bramwell Executive Services Ltd)
Top Santé (Emap Elan)
WeightWatchers Magazine (Castlebar Publishing)
You Are What You Eat (Brooklands Publishing)
Zest (National Magazine Company)

Index

◌ **Collins** need to know?

Look out for further titles in Collins' practical and accessible need to know? series.

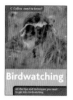 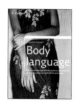 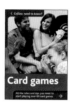 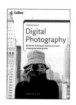

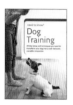 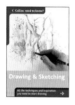 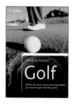 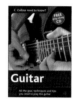 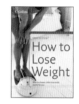

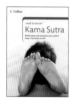 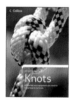   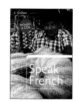

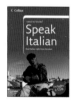 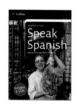 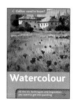 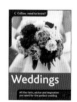

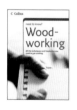 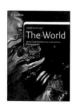 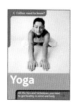 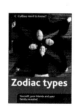 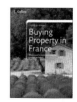

To order any of these titles, please telephone 0870 787 1732.

For further information on Collins books, please visit our website: www.collins.co.uk